"A big thank you to Josefowitz and Swallow for writing this much-needed
tion is among the most powerful methods for overcoming depression an
book provides a clear, step-by-step approach for using activity, exercis
mindfulness to rekindle motivation, energy, engagement, and enjoyment. I highly recommend it
for anyone who struggles with low mood!"

> —**Martin M. Antony, PhD, ABPP**, professor of psychology at Toronto Metropolitan
> University, and coauthor of *The Shyness and Social Anxiety Workbook* and *When
> Perfect Isn't Good Enough*

"This wonderful book offers clear, simple (but not simplistic!), manageable strategies for overcoming depression. Capitalizing on people's strengths, existent positive habits, and values, the book
naturally instills hope, motivation, and efficacy for change, while providing the scaffolding required
to effect that change. A must-read for clinicians and those living with depression."

> —**Christine Purdon, PhD, CPsych**, professor at the University of Waterloo, where
> she has taught cognitive behavioral therapy (CBT) for more than twenty-five years;
> and coauthor of *Overcoming Obsessive Thoughts*

"Depression is one of the most common mental health problems, and with COVID-19 has
increased. Two leading cognitive behavioral therapists offer important, evidence-based ways we
can help ourselves by seeing how we can get caught up in unhelpful loops of thinking and behavior, and then act to set up different loops that can lift us from depression. Full of clinical wisdom,
accessible, encouraging, and supportive, many depressed people will find key ideas and practices
to help them."

> —**Paul Gilbert, OBE**, author of *Overcoming Depression* and *The Compassionate Mind*

"Josefowitz and Swallow's focus on behavioral activation is comprehensive, ranging from methods
to increase social connections, strengthen motivation, and challenge avoidance patterns. They
emphasize practical, evidence-based steps to boost mood and cultivate happiness and well-being.
The authors' clinical acumen is evident in the many anecdotes and examples provided. This book
is replete with strategies and resources written in a straightforward and thought-provoking way,
and readers will come away with many ideas for the implementation and maintenance of effective
change."

> —**Deborah Dobson, PhD**, coauthor of *Evidence-Based Practice of Cognitive-Behavioral
> Therapy*; and **Keith Dobson, PhD**, coeditor of *Handbook of Cognitive-Behavioral
> Therapies*

"It has often been said that treatment is all about change, and with this workbook, Josefowitz and Swallow impressively demonstrate how change is possible in the context of the challenges of treating depression. They provide creative and original treatment strategies backed by sound research. These are presented in a persuasive and engaging style by two experienced and gifted therapists. This is recommended reading for all mental health professionals."

—**Karl O'Sullivan, FRCP(C), FRCPsych (UK)**, has held academic appointments in Ireland and Canada; and has published his psychiatric research in British, Canadian, and American journals

"This workbook is a critical tool for helping individuals learn effective strategies for overcoming depression. Using their extensive professional expertise, Josefowitz and Swallow bring effective, scientifically tested concepts to life by providing a clear, engaging, and highly practical guide to help readers identify and change 'mood-busting patterns.' This is a must-read for individuals who experience depression, and for the professionals who help them."

—**David J. A. Dozois, PhD**, professor, and director of the clinical psychology graduate program in the department of psychology at the University of Western Ontario

"This is an extremely important and useful resource for clinicians engaged in helping depressed individuals recover fully from their depression and move forward in their lives. Its focus on behavioral activation is a very helpful addition for all clinicians, especially those of us who have not focused enough on this key treatment approach. This volume is user-friendly, case-based, clear, and practical. It is written by experienced therapists/authors, and should be a valued go-to book for clinicians and clients."

—**Michael Rosenbluth, MD, FRCPC**, associate professor at the University of Toronto, and author of *Depression and Personality*

"This workbook is ideal for individuals who are depressed—as well as psychotherapists, social workers, and occupational therapists wanting to help their clients. It is a practical, goal-oriented guide that skillfully leverages an individual's strengths and values. It promotes clear, engaging problem-solving with a compassionate, mindful approach. The workbook offers diverse approaches to understanding behavioral activation and managing depression, empowering you in your journey toward a brighter future."

—**Nira Rittenberg, OT Reg (Ont)**, occupational therapist with thirty-five years in mental health, psychogeriatrics, and research expertise; and coauthor of *Dementia*

The
Behavioral Activation Workbook for Depression

Powerful Strategies to
Boost Your Mood & Build a Better Life

NINA JOSEFOWITZ, PHD

STEPHEN R. SWALLOW, PHD

New Harbinger Publications, Inc.

Publisher's Note

This publication is designed to provide accurate and authoritative information in regard to the subject matter covered. It is sold with the understanding that the publisher is not engaged in rendering psychological, financial, legal, or other professional services. If expert assistance or counseling is needed, the services of a competent professional should be sought.

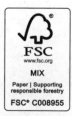

Printed in the United States of America

26   25   24

10   9   8   7   6   5   4   3   2   1   First Printing

To Novak Jankovic, the best NJ in my life
—NJ

To Wesley and Liam
—SRS

Contents

Foreword

Structured treatments for depression, introduced in the late 1970s, were a real boon for the long-term management of depression. Aaron Beck's cognitive therapy, Gerald Klerman's interpersonal psychotherapy, and Peter Lewinsohn's behavioral therapy provided vital points of departure from the generic intrapsychic models that dominated the therapeutic space. One chief advantage of these newer approaches was that they were explicit about the means required to help people recover from their illness and stay well. This was accomplished through detailed manuals describing each treatment session, tasks that engaged depression-specific mental and emotional content, and a commitment to empirical evaluation that could lead to further refinement based on identifying effective mechanisms of action.

In the over forty years since these manuals were made available, this strategy has paid dividends, generating strong empirical support for each approach and, perhaps more importantly, a clearer view of the underlying mechanisms that spur beneficial changes in the lives of people receiving precisely this type of care. Based on this literature, enrolling people in the larger project of counteracting the isolating, paralyzing, and punishing effects of depression is central to recovery. As long-standing cognitive therapists, Nina Josefowitz and Stephen Swallow understand this and their *Behavioral Activation Workbook* is an accessible and incisive guide that lays out how people can sign on to this project and reclaim their lives in the process. It might seem odd at first to link two practicing cognitive therapists with a book that is squarely focused on increasing environmental engagement. What about negative thoughts, cognitive distortions, or faulty beliefs providing the grist for the cognitive-treatment-of-depression mill? What is laudable about this book is that Nina and Stephen do not subscribe to a false binary in which one has to decide whether thoughts come first in changing behavior or whether behavior change is what changes people's beliefs. This is where the reader benefits from their cumulative clinical wisdom and expertise—a working premise of *The Behavioral Activation Workbook* is that the process is circular! Examining our thoughts can help us change how we act and, equally, changing how we act can allow us to update our beliefs. *The Behavioral Activation Workbook* lays out exactly how you can harness this wisdom for yourself.

This sounds good in principle, but how exactly does the reader jump in? What is most reassuring is that the authors' approach to unpacking behavioral activation—sometimes misconstrued as overly stoic and directive driven—emphasizes elements of compassion, self-affirmation, and exploration. These in turn establish a foundation for taking action that is validating and experience generating, regardless of the outcome.

Right from the outset, Nina and Stephen take a deep interest in the ways that depression shows up in people's lives. Not relying on a generic diagnosis, the reader is asked to describe how depression has limited their activity and engagement with the world. This is as much an effort to establish a baseline as it is to open the reader's eyes to how their world has shrunk and how this deficit keeps depression in place. The authors' emphasis on finding customized and personally relevant action plans continues to place the reader at the center of their efforts to either re-engage with activities that have been dropped or explore new ones. Still, finding activities that are effective and feasible is one thing; making them happen is another. In the face of challenging life circumstances, early life trauma, or harsh relationships, one can understand the reader's reluctance to wonder about the impact of small day-to-day changes in routine. Nina and Stephen remain undaunted. Their belief in the efficacy (as countless research studies have shown) and utility of starting small and building to bigger is one of the optimistic backbones of their workbook and serves to inspire the reader to explore the exercises laid out in each chapter.

One of the cardinal strengths of behavioral activation is that it helps the reader appreciate that when depression is present, thoughts and thinking patterns may abound, but their influence on taking action can be diminished. This is most evident when it comes to conducting behavioral experiments. Whether in the service of doing more of what used to provide a sense of mastery and connection, or breaking out of habits that support a constricted lifestyle, behavioral experiments let the reader dip a toe into the unknown. Yes, there will be thoughts at the outset such as *This won't make a difference* or *I already know how this will turn out*, but the beauty lies in seeing oneself go against the grain of the mind's predictions and doing it anyway. The authors provide a number of wonderful examples of this thrill of discovery, including my favorite—smiling at strangers and seeing what comes back your way.

The authors' vast clinical experience also shines through in the latter parts of the workbook, where issues of motivation and avoidance are addressed. To be honest, workbooks, digital apps, webinars, and other communication media have spotty records of adherence. The content in each of these channels may be high quality, but that does not guarantee sustained utilization. Nina and Stephen address this reality head-on. They ask the reader to identify the values they hold dear and then use these values to build motivation to engage in program activities. By identifying motivation-busting thoughts and beliefs, the reader is given a leg up on some of the ways they may undermine their own efforts. It also becomes easier for them to see how their symptoms stand in the way of living their values and why engaging with their symptoms makes perfect sense.

Today's marketplace is filled with books on depression that are popular and buzzworthy. If you are looking for a depression workbook that is user friendly, sensitive, and clinically astute, this is one of the best.

—Zindel V. Segal, PhD
Distinguished Professor of Psychology in Mood Disorders,
University of Toronto Scarborough

Introduction

Hello, and welcome to *The Behavioral Activation Workbook for Depression*. If you've picked up this book, it's probably because you—or possibly someone you care about—suffers from depression and you're looking for answers. Depression is really hard. Many of our clients say that the pain of depression is worse than any physical pain they've ever experienced. Over the years, the two of us have helped hundreds of clients overcome their depression, one step at a time. We've seen the pain of depression up close—but we also know that there is a way to push back on your depression and start to feel better.

When people get depressed, they lose their interest in doing things—they feel tired, apathetic, and unmotivated, so they stop doing things that once brought them pleasure, meaning, and fulfillment. But here's the rub: the less they do, the more tired, apathetic, unmotivated—and depressed—they feel. They get caught in a vicious, downward spiral of inactivity, low motivation, and ever-worsening mood. Sound familiar?

Many books on depression focus on changing thoughts and feelings. In this book, we're going to come at it from a slightly different angle. We're going to focus primarily on what you're *doing*. This approach is called "behavioral activation," and it has helped thousands and thousands of people just like you overcome their depression. It's an approach that is practical, easily understood, and very doable. Best of all, it works. A large body of scientific research has firmly established it as an effective treatment for depression (Richards et al. 2016).

Here's the idea: As you start to become more active, your mood improves—and as your mood improves, you become more motivated to engage in activities that make you feel even better. It's the exact opposite of what happens in depression. Behavioral activation is really about helping you get back into your life—and creating a better, more depression-resistant life in the process.

In this book, we'll guide you step by step through behavioral activation in a way that's very similar to what we do with our own clients. In part 1, we'll introduce you to the basic theory of behavioral activation and help you apply that theory to understanding your own feelings of depression. In part 2, we'll start identifying activities that we call the "building blocks" of a better, more depression-resistant life—and we'll show you how to start incorporating these activities into your own behavioral activation routine. In part 3, we'll tackle the problem of lethargy and low motivation. We'll introduce you to several powerful strategies for overcoming low motivation and for getting yourself going. Then in part 4, we'll give you tools for maintaining and building on the gains you've made, and for cultivating personal qualities like gratitude and compassion that set the stage for a life of true happiness and well-being.

As you read through the book, we want you to start applying the material right away. We'll often pause to give you a chance to reflect on and write about what you've learned. In addition, every chapter includes *What About You?* sections. These are exercises to help you apply the principles of behavioral activation to your own life. It's important to try them. The reality is that some of the exercises will help you more than others—but you won't know until you actually do them. We've posted all the worksheets and other supplementary material at http://www.newharbinger. com/52465. You'll find details at the back of the book—please feel free to download whatever you need to help you on your behavioral activation journey.

We've tried to keep the tone of this workbook informal and friendly. We've even shared a few illustrations from our own personal lives. We hope you'll find that helpful.

Overcoming depression is not easy, and it can take some time. But there *is* hope. If you feel a bit daunted at the prospect of facing down your depression, don't worry. We're going to take you through it one step at a time. We believe you can do it! So let's get started…

PART ONE

Foundations of
Behavioral Activation

CHAPTER 1

Understand Your Depression— and Discover a Way Out

Do you feel sad, overwhelmed, or hopeless? Do you lack energy and have trouble getting going? Have you lost interest in activities you used to enjoy or do you find it hard to concentrate? If so, you may be suffering from depression. It's important to know that you aren't alone, and that there *is* hope for recovery. If you feel stuck in a negative cycle of low mood, lack of motivation, and just not caring about life anymore, this workbook can help you find your way out.

Millions of people all over the world—people from every racial, cultural, socioeconomic background, religion, age, gender, and sexual orientation—live with the pain of depression. Whether your depression is mild, severe, or somewhere in between, we want to introduce you to a very powerful approach for pushing back on your depression and creating a better, more depression-resistant life. It's an approach called "behavioral activation."

Hundreds of research studies support the effectiveness of behavioral activation in treating depression. We've also seen the benefits of using behavioral activation in our own work with clients over the years, so we think there's a very good chance that behavioral activation will also help you. But please don't take our word for it. We hope you'll approach this workbook as an experiment. Test it out for yourself. See if it works. We think you'll find that it's well worth the effort.

We'll dive a little deeper into behavioral activation later in this chapter. But first, we're going to help you understand your own depression a little better.

Know Your Symptoms of Depression

For some people, depression seems to come out of nowhere. For others, major losses, negative life events, or multiple daily difficulties trigger their depression. No matter how your depression may have started, the suffering it causes is very real. Depression can affect nearly every area of your life—physical, emotional, mental, social, and spiritual. So what exactly does it mean to be depressed? Let's take a closer look.

Everyone experiences depression a little differently. Here is a list of some of the most common symptoms. Have a look through and see how many of these may apply to you.

- Feeling sad, down, or depressed

- Decreased interest in or enjoyment from most activities

- Feeling hopeless or discouraged about the future

- Feeling like a failure

- Feeling guilty and worthless

- Crying more than usual

- Feeling irritated or annoyed

- Wanting to avoid being with other people

- Decreased or increased appetite for food; weight loss (without dieting) or weight gain

- Having less energy and being more tired than usual

- Finding it difficult to get going

- Finding it difficult to concentrate or make decisions

Most of us have some of these symptoms from time to time. That's just a normal part of life. But if you've been experiencing many of these symptoms for most of the day, for at least a couple of weeks at a time, there's a reasonably good chance that you are suffering from depression.

When people are depressed, it's not uncommon for them to have recurrent thoughts of death or dying. Some people may even have a plan to end their lives. If this is how depression is affecting you—especially if you feel you may act on your thoughts or if you have a specific plan to harm yourself or end your life—it's important to contact your family physician or a mental health professional to discuss your feelings. If you're in crisis, talk to someone or call a local distress line right away. Googling "suicide helpline" will provide resources in your area.

Meet Maya

In this workbook, we're going to focus on two clients, Maya and Ed. From time to time, we'll also include examples of other clients. Maya is a composite of many of the clients Nina has treated, and Ed is a composite of many of Stephen's clients. You'll meet Ed a bit later. None of the clients in this book are our actual clients, but are based on a combination of clients we have known.

Maya is a thirty-eight-year-old high school teacher. Her husband left her six years ago, and she has two young children at home, Vanie (age eight) and Jaco (age six). Maya had been depressed in the past but felt that she had gotten over it. She became depressed again about a year after her mother's death. Her mother had been sick for a few years before her death, and Maya was very involved in her mother's care during the last year of her life.

Maya told Nina that her depression was getting worse—that she was weepy and felt exhausted, and that if she wasn't at work she spent a lot of the day doing nothing. She felt that she was a useless mother and no longer really enjoyed being with her children. Her long-term boyfriend had cheated on her and although she had ended the relationship, she was lonely and missed him. Over the past year she had gained twenty pounds and really disliked how she looked. She felt pretty hopeless about anything in her life getting better.

When Maya looked at the list of symptoms of depression, she realized that many of them applied to her. She found it somewhat comforting to know she was not alone, and that many other people struggled with experiences similar to hers.

What About You?

Throughout this book we have exercises that we call "What About You?" These exercises are an important opportunity to apply what we've covered in the chapter to your own life. We hope you will try them—they will help you get more out of the book.

Look back at the list of symptoms of depression. Then, on the *My Symptoms of Depression* worksheet, list all the symptoms that apply to you. You can add any additional symptoms that may be a part of your depression. After you write down your symptoms, see if you can rate the severity of each symptom. Severity is a combination of how often you experience the symptom as well as its strength. A rating of 1 means the symptom is very mild, and a 10 means the symptom is very severe.

My Symptoms of Depression	
Symptom	Severity 1 (very mild) to 10 (very severe)

Understand Your Mood-Busting Cycle

If you are depressed, you probably know the feeling of being enveloped in a big cloud of negativity. This negativity is actually made up of negative feelings, thoughts, and behaviors. For example, when you are depressed, you *feel* sad, hopeless, tired, and unmotivated. These feelings are associated with negative, demotivating *thoughts* such as *Everything is too hard*; *Nothing matters*; *No one cares about me*; *I don't matter*; or *Nothing will ever get better*. These thoughts and feelings lead to changes in your behavior. For example, you may sleep more, exercise less, see friends and family less often, do less at work, and ignore your hobbies. When depressed, people generally tend to be less active, to withdraw from activities they previously enjoyed, and to avoid facing their problems. This illustration shows how the feelings and thoughts associated with depression negatively impact behavior.

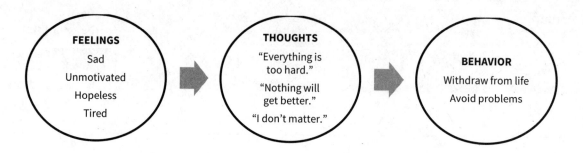

Figure 1.1: Depression Has a Negative Impact on Behavior

However, this model is only half the puzzle. The piece that's missing—and it's a really important piece—is that not only do our depressed feelings and thoughts cause us to withdraw from life, but *when we withdraw from life and avoid our problems, we become even more depressed.*

We italicized that point to be sure you would stop and notice it—and we're even going to repeat it below.

Withdraw from Life + Avoid Problems = Become More Depressed

Take a look at this illustration, and think about how it applies to you.

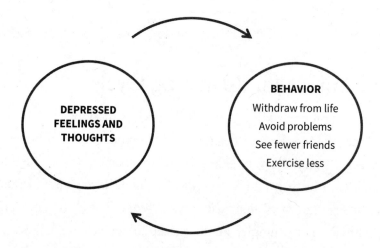

Figure 1.2: Behavior Maintains the Vicious Cycle of Depression

Mood-Busting Behaviors

Let's look at some specific examples of the things we tend to do when we're depressed. We call these "mood-busting behaviors" because they're really good at undermining any positive feelings we may be having, and dragging us down into depression. You will see that there is a great deal of overlap in these categories. That's okay. This list is not exhaustive—it's just meant to get you thinking about mood-busting behaviors.

Avoiding or decreasing social contact. This may involve seeing family, friends, or work colleagues less often. People often engage in this kind of mood-busting behavior because it can feel safer or easier to be home alone.

Avoiding or decreasing activities that bring you enjoyment or pleasure. This may involve listening less frequently to good music, neglecting hobbies you enjoy, or giving up your morning visits to the coffee shop.

Avoiding or decreasing activities that bring you a sense of accomplishment or mastery. This may involve letting go of everyday tasks you are good at, such as cooking or fixing things—or giving up on bigger goals like finishing school or learning a new skill.

Avoiding or decreasing activities that provide you with a sense of meaning or purpose. This may involve giving up activities that are consistent with your values, like volunteer work, or caring for a child, family member, friend, or pet.

Avoiding or decreasing activities that are good for your health. This may involve decreasing how much you exercise, slipping into irregular sleeping patterns, or developing unhealthy eating habits.

Increasing activities that make you feel good initially but are not healthy in the long run. This may involve increasing how much you drink alcohol, use drugs, gamble, binge-watch TV, or use the internet/social media.

Avoiding or procrastinating. This involves sidestepping or putting off important tasks or situations that seem difficult, uncomfortable, or overwhelming in some way.

As you look at this list of behaviors, does it start to make sense to you why we get so stuck in our depression? As we disengage from life and start using unhelpful coping strategies, our lives get worse and worse and our stress increases. As we withdraw from friends and family, we feel more alone. Avoiding our problems tends to make them worse. And if we disrupt sleep and eating routines we tend to feel even less well. The net result? We get caught in a vicious cycle in which we do less and less of the things that make us happy, and more and more of the things that make us miserable—and our depression gets worse and worse.

Let's take a look at how Maya's behavior contributed to her vicious cycle of depression. Maya told Nina that since her mother's illness, she was always tired and had started lying down and resting as much as she could. She just didn't feel like doing anything. In the past when her ex-husband had the children on weekends she used to go out to movies or dinner with friends or her boyfriend. Now she stayed home most of the time. She had also stopped swimming at the local pool. Because she was home so much, she had started drinking more alcohol than usual. She also spent more time on social media and browsing the internet. Maya used to make home-cooked meals that her kids particularly liked, and sometimes she would bake cookies. She realized she had not done either of those things since she became depressed. Maya sighed and said that she felt as if she had withdrawn from life.

Maya was embarrassed to admit that she was so stressed about money that she had not yet filed the taxes on her mother's estate and was avoiding calling the accountant. She was also pro-crastinating on making a budget and paying bills. She smiled ruefully at Nina as she said, "Of course, the more I procrastinate, the more I worry!"

Maya had always thought that her depression had caused her to stop doing many of her previous activities. But now she was starting to wonder if her withdrawal and her avoidance of these activities were actually contributing to her depression.

What About You?

Take a moment to reflect on your own mood-busting behavior, then complete the *My Mood-Busting Behaviors* worksheet that follows. Try to include examples from your own life for any category that is relevant for you.

My Mood-Busting Behaviors	
Type of mood-busting behavior	**Examples from my life**
Avoiding or decreasing social contact	
Avoiding or decreasing activities that bring me enjoyment or pleasure	
Avoiding or decreasing activities that bring me a sense of mastery or accomplishment	
Avoiding or decreasing activities that bring me a sense of meaning or purpose	
Avoiding or decreasing activities that are good for my health	
Increasing activities that make me feel good initially, but are not healthy long-term	
Avoiding facing my problems or procrastination on important tasks	
Other mood-busting behaviors (specify)	

The Mood-Boosting Cycle of Behavioral Activation

How does behavioral activation fit into all of this? Earlier we saw that our feelings of depression and our mood-busting behavior interact in a vicious cycle. What this means is that not only can our mood-busting behavior keep the cycle of depression going, but—on a much more encouraging note—changing our behavior can interrupt and even reverse the vicious cycle of depression. *Changing our behavior can change our mood.* Take a moment to think about this. It's really important.

> *Change Your Behavior to Change Your Mood*

We are going to help you change the behavior that fuels your depression. And the good news is that as you change your mood-busting behavior and begin to engage in more of what we call "mood-boosting behavior," you will start to feel less depressed and more motivated, and you will have fewer of those negative thoughts that bring you down. In short, you will create a positive cycle of increased activity and improved mood which, over time, will result in a happier, more fulfilling, more depression-resistant life.

Certain types of activities are particularly effective at boosting our mood and countering the negativity of depression. We refer to these activities as the building blocks of a good, depression-resistant life. They include the following:

- activities that bring us enjoyment or pleasure

- activities that promote physical activity

- activities that involve social connections

- activities that resonate with our personal values

- activities that foster a sense of mastery and accomplishment

- activities that help us face and solve our problems

Using the tools of behavioral activation, we're going to help you find the combination of activities that works best for you and will give your mood the biggest boost. As you start to engage in more and more mood-boosting behavior, your life will begin to change. Your mood will lift. You'll begin to feel better about yourself and your confidence will increase. It will begin to feel easier to face and find solutions to your problems. This illustration shows the mood-boosting cycle of behavioral activation.

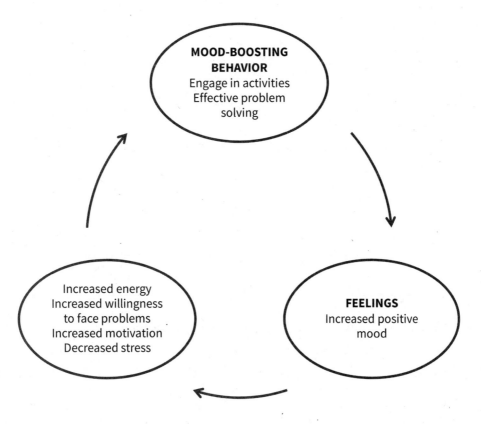

Figure 1.3: The Mood-Boosting Cycle of Behavioural Activation

It won't happen all at once, and it certainly won't be easy. When you're depressed, it can be really hard to even think of doing any of the mood-boosting activities we just mentioned, even if you know they may help. That's okay. We're going to show you how to introduce these activities into your life in a way that will make them feel doable and sustainable. We believe you can do it!

What About You?

We are going to spend a lot of time in this book helping you build your personal toolkit of mood-boosting behaviors. It may be a bit too early to start, but are you thinking about any specific mood-boosting activities you may want to begin incorporating into your life right away? Write them down here.

_____

_____

_____

What was it like to think of adding mood-boosting activities to your life? Take a moment to reflect—and perhaps to jot down your thoughts.

_____

_____

_____

Were you able to come up with some ideas for mood-boosting activities that you'd like to incorporate into your life? You can get a head start on your behavioral activation work by picking one activity from your list and then finding time to do it. Congratulations! This will be your first step in behavioral activation.

If you had difficulty thinking of any mood-boosting behaviors, don't worry. Many people who struggle with depression find this hard. Throughout this book we'll provide you with tools to help you find activities that will break your vicious cycle of depression and help create a positive cycle of behavioral activation and improved mood.

Why We Like Behavioral Activation

Both of us have used behavioral activation for many years in our work with clients suffering from depression. We have also used it in our own lives. We have seen it work, and we think it can work for you. But there are a few other reasons for our enthusiasm for behavioral activation.

It's Doable

The reality is, we have relatively little direct control over our feelings and physical sensations. It's pretty hard to just drum up feelings of happiness or shake off feelings of guilt, hopelessness, or fatigue. We also don't have that much control over our thinking—it's hard, if not impossible, to keep negative thoughts from popping into our heads. By contrast, we generally have more control over what we do. Making changes in our behavior—especially when we take it in small steps—is definitely more doable than changing how we feel or how we think.

It's Positive and Present-Oriented

Many people who are depressed have had very hard lives—difficult childhoods; major losses; experiences of abandonment, prejudice, or abuse; or other forms of trauma or adversity. Talking about and processing these experiences with a therapist is often very helpful. Behavioral activation, however, focuses on what we can do today—in the here and now—to create as good a life for ourselves as possible and to push back on our depression. We think this is an intrinsically positive, life-affirming approach to feeling better.

Others may be experiencing serious difficulties right now—difficulties that have either triggered their depression or made it worse. Perhaps you (or a loved one) are dealing with a frightening health issue, being bullied or disrespected at school or work, or having financial struggles, relationship problems, or social problems. Behavioral activation can help you stay strong and resilient in the face of these types of challenges—and may even give you tools for addressing some of the problems you're encountering (see chapter 7).

If you've been exposed to hurtful experiences in your life, especially if they happened in your childhood, you may feel that you don't matter, and that you don't deserve to be happy. If this is true for you, it may be extra hard to start taking steps toward feeling better. One of the very encouraging messages of behavioral activation is that no matter who you are, or what experiences you have had in your life, you are a valuable person whose happiness and well-being are important. As you work your way through this book, we hope you'll be open to valuing yourself and seeing the importance of creating a good and happy life for yourself. It will take some courage, but it's important.

It's Based on Research

The verdict is in: behavioral activation really works. Hundreds of studies have documented its effectiveness in the treatment of depression. The evidence is so solid that after considering all of the research, the practice guidelines of psychological and psychiatric associations from all over the world have recognized behavioral activation as an effective evidence-based treatment for depression (for example, United States: American Psychological Association, 2019; Australia and New Zealand: Malhi et al., 2021; Great Britain: National Institute for Health and Care Excellence (NICE), 2022; Canada: Parikh et al., 2016). This means that everything we are going to tell you is backed by research.

What's Next?

In this chapter we've introduced you to behavioral activation as an effective way to break and reverse the vicious cycle of depression. As you reflect on this chapter, what resonated most strongly with you?

_____

_____

_____

How could you apply what we covered in this chapter to your life right now?

_____

_____

_____

In the next chapter, we're going to focus on the relationship between *your* patterns of behavior and *your* depression. We'll give you a framework for understanding the ways in which your behavior is maintaining your depression, and show you how to use what you discover to start feeling better.

CHAPTER 2

Identify Your Mood-Busting Patterns

Before we start considering how you can change your behavior to improve your mood, we need to have a clearer sense of how depression is affecting your current behavior. In this chapter we're going to take stock of how your behavior has changed since you became depressed and look at how these changes are affecting your mood. We'll then help you find patterns in your own daily activities that you can use to break your cycle of depression. We'll be using Ed as an illustration. Let's start by introducing him to you.

Meet Ed

Ed—a composite of Stephen's depressed clients—is a twenty-seven-year-old skilled carpenter. He's married to Judy, and together they have a three-year-old son, Alex. When he came for treatment, Ed had been off work for two years due to severe pain, numbness, and weakness in his right hand and wrist from repetitive strain. The doctors suspected nerve damage, but none of the various tests found anything conclusive.

Prior to being injured, Ed worked long hours and earned a very good living. He was happy spending time with his wife and loved roughhousing with his son. He enjoyed hanging out with his coworkers, both on the job site and occasionally at the local pub.

Ed and his wife often invited their family or friends over on weekends. Ed would grill hamburgers and sausages. During the winter, he played ice hockey with a group of high school buddies. During the summer, he played soccer and sometimes golf. When Ed first began having hand and wrist pain, he saw a variety of doctors and physiotherapists. Nothing helped. Ed became more and more discouraged. He was receiving compensation payments, but they were a fraction of what he earned at work. He worried about his ability to provide for his family. Ed had grown up in a family where being a hard worker was a source of great pride and honor. He was embarrassed and ashamed not to be working.

As Ed's mood worsened, he stopped doing a lot of the activities he used to enjoy. He spent his days watching game shows and sports reruns on TV. Ice hockey was out—he could no longer hold a hockey stick well enough to play. Ed began to avoid seeing friends and family members because he felt so embarrassed about not working. He was worried they would think he was "milking the system." He started snacking more and drinking more beer to pass the time at home. As a result, he gained weight. He felt uncomfortable about how his body had changed. His mood grew worse and worse. He did not like the person he had become. To Ed, the future seemed hopeless and bleak.

Identify What's Changed

To clearly understand how depression is affecting your behavior—and to get ideas for potential mood-boosting activities—it's important to be aware of how your activities have changed since becoming depressed. Over the years, we have found that the *Change in My Activities* worksheet (see below) is a good way for people to identify how depression has impacted their activities. You can use it to compare your activities before you became depressed to your activities now. If you have been depressed for a long time, you can compare your current activities to a time when you felt relatively better. Remember, we're focusing here on how your depression has changed what you *do*—not how you feel. This may be a new way of looking at depression for you, but let's give it a try.

We completed the *Changes in My Activities* worksheet with examples from Ed's life to show you how to use it. You will see there is quite a bit of overlap in Ed's responses to the different categories—that's pretty normal. After looking at Ed's responses, take some time to fill in your own.

Changes in My Activities	
Life events associated with the onset of my depression (if any)	
Ed: I developed pain, numbness, and weakness in my right hand and wrist, and had to stop working. Me:	
Type of activities	**How my activities have changed since the onset of my depression**
Activities I enjoy and/or that give me a sense of accomplishment	Increased: Watching sports shows; playing video games; hanging out with my son Decreased: Playing hockey and soccer with the guys; socializing with my family and work buddies; washing my car; fixing things around the house; going to work; walking with my wife
	Me
Activities I don't enjoy	Increased: Spending time alone; watching daytime TV Decreased: Driving to work in the winter
	Me

Type of activities	How my activities have changed since the onset of my depression
Physical exercise	Increased: None Decreased: Playing hockey and soccer regularly; occasional golf game; going for walks with my wife
	Me
Spending time with friends	Increased: Hanging out with my online gaming buddies Decreased: Going to the pub with work friends; hanging out with buddies after hockey and soccer games; BBQs in our home; going to friends' homes
	Me
Spending time with family	Increased: Having father-son time with Alex Decreased: Having family over for BBQs; going on date night with my wife; roughhousing with Alex
	Me:

Type of activities	How my activities have changed since the onset of my depression
Leisure or hobbies	Increased: Video games Decreased: Golfing with buddies; fooling around with my car
	Me:
Smoking, eating patterns, alcohol or drug use	Increased: Eating chips and cookies; drinking beer during the day Decreased: None
	Me
Routines related to sleeping	Increased: Staying up late and snacking in front of the TV Decreased: Going to bed with my wife; getting up when Alex wakes up
	Me
Other ways I cope	Increased: Video games Decreased: None
	Me

People have a variety of reactions to completing this worksheet. Sometimes they feel overwhelmed as they take a hard look at their lives. Other people may feel a sense of relief as their depression starts to make more sense. When Ed completed the worksheet, he was really struck by all the ways his life had changed since his injury. He had not even been aware of some of the changes; others he had not really considered to be all that significant. He began to see that many of these changes were actually feeding back into his depression. This was a new perspective for Ed.

Whatever your reaction, it takes courage to take a close look at your life and complete the worksheet. Understanding the relationship between your activities and your depression is an important step in feeling better.

Take a moment to reflect on the worksheet. What did you learn about your own behavior and the way it has changed since becoming depressed?

_____

_____

_____

_____

_____

Track Your Daily Activities

We're now going to take a closer look at how your activities are affecting your moods. To do this, we'd like to encourage you to start tracking your activities *and* your moods throughout the day. This will give you some idea of how your mood may fluctuate over the course of each day. But very importantly, it will also provide information on how your activities—what you do or don't do—are affecting how you feel.

When you are depressed, it can feel as if your depression is an unchanging negative cloud that hangs over you. However, when you look at your day more closely, you'll often discover that your mood actually fluctuates more than you might have thought. Detecting even small changes in your mood can be important. You may learn, for example, that you feel better at certain times of the day than at others. You may also discover that you feel better after engaging in certain activities than you do after others.

You can use the *Daily Activities* worksheet (see below) to track which activities are associated with feeling better and which activities are associated with a lower mood. We are then going to use this information to identify activities that can help you feel better. Everyone is different—so you'll need to find the combination and the type of mood-boosting activities that work best for you.

The *Daily Activities* worksheet tracks what you do every hour of the day and asks you to rate your mood on a scale from 1 to 10. A rating of 1 means that you feel as low and depressed as you've ever felt, and a rating of 10 means you feel as good as you've ever felt. If you engaged in more than one activity per hour, just jot down the two most important ones, or use one word to capture what you did—for example, "errands."

Before you fill out your own *Daily Activities* worksheet, take a look at how Maya completed hers. You can use it as a guide. For another example, you can have a look at Ed's *Daily Activities* worksheet, available for download.

	Maya's Daily Activities						
	1 (very depressed) to 10 (very happy)						
Time	Monday	Tuesday	Wednesday	Thursday	Friday	Saturday	Sunday
6:00 a.m.	Lay in bed (1)			Lay in bed (1)			
7:00 a.m.	Lay in bed (1)	Lay in bed (1)		Got up on time (3)	Woke up–lay in bed (1)		
8:00 a.m.	Started breakfast for kids (2) Got kids ready for school (2)	Started breakfast for kids (2) Got kids ready for school (3)	Late–breakfast for kids, got kids ready for school (1)	Breakfast for kids (4) Got kids ready for school (2)			
9:00 a.m.	Dropped kids off at school, drove to work (3)	Dropped kids off at school, drove to work (3)	Took kids to school, drove to work (2)	Took kids to school, drove to work (4)			Woke up (1)
10:00 a.m.	Taught (3)	Taught (3)	Assembly (4)	Taught (4)	Taught (4)	Lay in bed, then breakfast (2)	Lay in bed, breakfast (2)
11:00 a.m.	Taught (3)	Taught (4)	Taught (4)	Professional development course (5)	Taught (3)	Cleaned house, laundry (4)	Returned email, helped a friend of mother's who can't drive (5)
12:00 p.m.	Lunch at desk and admin work (2)	Lunch with colleague (6)	Lunch with same colleague (5)	Lunch at desk, admin work (2)	Lunch at desk and walked with colleague (5)	Errands, food shopping – bumped into friend from swimming and chatted (5)	Visited mother's friend and did errands (6)
1:00 p.m.	Taught (3)	Taught (5)	Gave students a test (4)	Taught (3)	Taught (5)	Napped (3)	Visited with mother's friend and did errands (6)
2:00 p.m.	Spare period–walked (4)	Spare period–prepared for next day (5)	Spare period–graded papers (5)	Taught (3)	Spare period–graded papers (5)	Napped (3)	Visited with mother's friend and did errands (6)

Time	Monday	Tuesday	Wednesday	Thursday	Friday	Saturday	Sunday
3:00 p.m.	Spare period—graded homework (5)	Spare period—graded homework (3)	Taught (5)	Met with colleagues to discuss curriculum changes (4)	Taught (3)	Graded papers (4)	Drove home, napped (4)
4:00 p.m.	Picked up kids from school (5)	Picked up kids from school (5)	Picked up kids, stopped for ice cream (6)	Picked up kids (5)	Picked up kids and dropped them off at their father's house (3)	Cooked food for potluck dinner with friends (6)	Emails and texting friends (6)
5:00 p.m.	Made dinner Homework with kids (4)	Made dinner Tried to do banking related to mother (2)	Board games with the kids (5)	Homework with son (5)	Drove home, social media (3)	Got ready for the evening (4)	Prepared for classes (3)
6:00 p.m.	Dinner with kids (4)	Dinner alone (2)	Dinner with kids (5)	Dinner with kids (4)	Social media (2)	Dinner with a few friends (5)	Social media (3)
7:00 p.m.	TV with kids (7)	Laundry (3)	Homework with the kids (4)	Homework with son—we fought (2)	Social media (2)	Dinner with friends (6)	Social media (3)
8:00 p.m.	Bedtime with kids (5)	Bedtime with kids (3)	Bedtime with kids (5)	Bedtime with kids (4)	Texted with a couple of friends—group chat (6)	Dinner with friends (6)	Social media (3)
9:00 p.m.	Social media (2)	Social media (3)	Cleaned kitchen, laundry, housework (5)	Tried to do a budget (1)	Social media (3)	Dinner with friends (6)	Social media (3)
10:00 p.m.	Talked to aunt who called (8)	Social media (2)	Read emails, read a magazine (4)	Tried to do budget (1)	Social media (2)	Home, tidied up kitchen, played video game (6)	Bed (3)
11:00 p.m.	Social media (1)	Social media (2)	Got ready for bed and took a bath (4)	Social media (1)	Netflix movie (6)	Video game, got ready for bed (6)	
12:00 a.m.	Sleep	Sleep	Sleep	Sleep	Sleep	Sleep	

Maya thought that completing her *Daily Activities* worksheet would be hard and take a lot of time, but it took only a few minutes each day to jot down her activities and rate her mood. She actually enjoyed doing it as she felt she was starting to work on her depression.

When Maya looked at her *Daily Activities* worksheet she was surprised at how much her mood fluctuated over the week. She felt as if she was always down, but there was actually quite a lot of variation.

Maya had always assumed that being depressed was causing her to lack the energy and enthusiasm for doing the things she used to like to do. After completing the *Daily Activities* worksheet, she realized that staying home, and not doing what she used to enjoy, was actually feeding into her depression and her lack of energy. For Maya, this was an important insight.

What About You?

It's time for you to begin tracking your daily activities and discovering more about the relationship between what you do and how you feel.

Recording your activities hour by hour every day may feel a bit daunting. We get that. So just start by recording your activities for one day—today. Please keep in mind that it doesn't have to be done perfectly! Some people find it easier to record their activities on an hour-by-hour basis. Others prefer to do it all at once—say at the end of the day. Do whatever works best for you. Don't forget to record and rate your mood beside each activity. We think you'll find it pretty interesting.

Time	Monday	Tuesday	Wednesday	Thursday	Friday	Saturday	Sunday
My Daily Activities **1 (very depressed) to 10 (very happy)**							
6:00 a.m.							
7:00 a.m.							
8:00 a.m.							
9:00 a.m.							
10:00 a.m.							
11:00 a.m.							

Time	Monday	Tuesday	Wednesday	Thursday	Friday	Saturday	Sunday
12:00 p.m.							
1:00 p.m.							
2:00 p.m.							
3:00 p.m.							
4:00 p.m.							
5:00 p.m.							

Time	Monday	Tuesday	Wednesday	Thursday	Friday	Saturday	Sunday
6:00 p.m.							
7:00 p.m.							
8:00 p.m.							
9:00 p.m.							
10:00 p.m.							
11:00 p.m.							
12:00 a.m.							

Explore Your Patterns

Once you've started completing the *Daily Activities* worksheet, you can begin looking for patterns. Recording your activities and your moods for even a single day can help you begin to notice activities that are associated with boosts in your mood and other activities that seem to be associated with lower moods. As you gather more information from day to day, you'll see more and more of these connections. We're going to use this information to help you make a mood-boosting plan.

Drawing on information from your *Daily Activities* worksheet, use the questions in the *Patterns in My Life* worksheet below to help you learn how your pattern of activities is connected to your moods. Some of the questions assume that you've completed the *Daily Activities* for the whole week. Don't worry if this is not the case. Just work with what you have.

We've answered each question with examples from Maya's *Daily Activities* worksheet. We've left space for you to record your answers as well.

Patterns in My Life	
What activities boost my mood?	Maya: I feel better when I'm spending time with friends and other people; spending fun time with my kids; taking a walk; and playing video games and movies. I also feel better at school than I expected.
	Me:
What activities lower my mood?	Maya: I spend a lot of time on social media, and I feel worse afterward. I also get really depressed when I try to pay my bills and start to make a budget.
	Me:

What are the best times of the day for me?	Maya: Lunchtimes at work are pretty good, especially if I do something with a friend or don't just stay at my desk.
	Me:
What are the worst times of the day for me?	Maya: Mornings are really hard for me—I wake up early and toss and turn. I think about my mother and feel sorry for myself. Evenings are also hard—I feel sad and empty after spending time on social media.
	Me:
What are the best days of the week for me?	Maya: Sunday afternoons are good—I usually do errands and sometimes I visit my mother's friend.
	Me:
What are the worst days of the week for me?	Maya: Sunday evenings are pretty bad—I'm sort of dreading going back to work on Monday.
	Me:

Did you notice any patterns? Were you able to identify any activities that seem to either boost your mood or bust your mood? If you were able to track your activities over the course of the whole week, did you notice any patterns? Some people, for example, find that weekends are quite a bit different from weekdays. Think about your own patterns, and use the space below to reflect on what you learned.

_____

_____

_____

_____

_____

_____

_____

_____

Even if you completed the *Daily Activities* worksheet for only a couple of days, it will still give you important information that you can use to put together an effective behavioral activation plan. We're curious what you will find.

Some people really don't like using the *Daily Activities* worksheet. If that's you—no problem. You can also try writing your activities into a diary or dictating them into your smartphone. You can then use the questions in the *Patterns in My Life* worksheet to examine what you recorded. Other people have found different ways that work for them. The real goal here is to discover the patterns between your activities and your mood. With that information in hand, we can help you start to do more of what makes you feel better and find ways to change your low mood times.

What's Next?

In this chapter we've gotten a bit more personal—we explored the relationship between your activities and your moods. As you think over the chapter, what has been important to you?

_____

_____

_____

_____

_____

_____

How can you incorporate what you learned into your daily life?

_____

_____

_____

_____

_____

_____

In the next section of this workbook, we'll look at a range of mood-boosting activities that constitute the building blocks of a happy, meaningful, and depression-resistant life. The next chapter focuses on identifying activities that may bring you some enjoyment or pleasure. We'll also show you how to develop a really effective behavioral activation plan—one that you can implement successfully and then stick with. Let's get going!

PART TWO

Building Blocks for Behavioral Activation

CHAPTER 3

Find What You Enjoy, Make a Plan, and Get Started!

Creating a happy, meaningful, depression-resistant life doesn't happen all at once. We're going to take it one step at a time. The first building block for pushing back on your depression involves adding activities to your life that you enjoy—even a little bit—or that you find pleasurable. We call these your "pleasurable" mood-boosting behaviors. We're going to look at three strategies to help you identify these activities.

Start with What's Already Working

A good place to start is to find activities you are already doing that boost your mood, even a little, by bringing you some enjoyment or pleasure—and then do them more often. Either look over your *Daily Activities* worksheet, or, if you didn't complete that worksheet, notice what you were doing and who you were with when your mood was even a little bit better.

Maya used her *Daily Activities* worksheet (see chapter 2) to identify enjoyable activities that were associated with her better moods. These included playing board games with her children; having lunch with a colleague; going for a walk at lunch; chatting with a friend from swimming; cooking; having dinner with friends; and doing errands with her mother's friend. Maya was surprised at how much her mood varied over the week. She chose three activities that she would like to do again—and even do more often this coming week:

1. Play board games with my children.

2. Have lunch again with a colleague—either the same colleague or a different one.

3. On the weekend do errands and get out of the house.

It can be helpful before you look at your own life to practice seeing patterns and thinking about what activities someone else could add to their life. You'll find Ed's *Daily Activities* worksheet online. See if you can identify activities that Ed could continue doing to boost his mood.

What About You?

Now it's time to focus on you. You can either look over your *Daily Activities* worksheet or think of what you were doing this past week that you enjoyed and that made you feel a bit better—even if just a little. Next, choose three activities that you would like to continue doing or maybe even do a little more often.

1. _____

2. _____

3. _____

You just took an important first step in feeling better. Let's build on it.

Do What You Used to Enjoy

Another way to identify pleasurable mood-boosting activities is to start doing some of the activities you used to enjoy before you became depressed but have stopped doing. The *Changes in My Activities* worksheet from chapter 2 can help you identify these activities. Even if you have been depressed for a long time, there has probably been a period when you felt somewhat better. Think back to that time and the activities you enjoyed. Even if you can no longer do what you used to like, is it possible to do something similar?

When Ed looked at his *Changes in My Activities* worksheet he immediately commented that he missed exercising—especially playing hockey and going for walks with his wife. Ed grinned sheepishly as he looked at the worksheet and said it would be nice to go out with his wife for dinner sometimes. He also missed his buddies—he hadn't seen his work friends or his hockey or soccer buddies in a long time. He paused and said, "When I think of it, I could have some family or old friends over for a barbecue." Ed made a list of three activities that he missed doing. These included having friends over for a barbecue; going for a walk with his wife; and going to a restaurant with his wife.

Let's look at another example. Eva was being sexually harassed by her boss. There were constant comments about her body, how her boss wished he was twenty years younger, and how lucky her husband was to have such a "hot" wife. Eva tried to ignore the comments, but they became more and more frequent. Over the past few months, Eva had started to become depressed. She wasn't sure how to handle the sexual harassment and wanted to take her time thinking about what she could do. She did know that she wanted to take better care of herself so that she could stay strong and not fall into a depression. Eva made a list of the activities she used to enjoy but had stopped doing because she was so overwhelmed by her boss's behavior. She decided to start seeing some of her closest girlfriends again, and to start having some "me" time during which she worked on arts and crafts that she had previously enjoyed.

What About You?

Since you became depressed, what previously enjoyed activities have you stopped engaging in? Which of those activities would make good mood boosters? To help you with this, we're going to ask you a few questions. Write down your answer to each question. Different questions may have the same answer.

Which activity do you think would make the biggest difference to your life if you started doing it again?

_____

Which activity would you like to start doing again?

_____

Which activities do you miss the most?

_____

Which activity would a good friend or caring family member suggest you start doing again?

_____

Look over your answers, and choose three activities you might want to add to your life.

1. _____

2. _____

3. _____

Take some time to reflect on the exercises you just completed. What was it like to start thinking about engaging in some of the activities you used to enjoy? Were these the same activities that came to mind when you reflected on activities that were already working, or were they different? Write down your thoughts here.

_____

_____

_____

_____

_____

Find Some Enjoyable Activities

When people are depressed it can be really hard for them to come up with ideas for activities they might find enjoyable. We've often found it helpful to ask our depressed clients to look over lists of activities that other people generally find enjoyable and then to see if they can find a few that they may be tempted to try for themselves. We usually ask our clients to look for activities they don't generally do, but which they think they might enjoy—even just a little bit. If they struggle with this, we suggest they look for activities from the list that they may have enjoyed before becoming depressed.

There are literally thousands of activities that people may find enjoyable. Everyone is different but anything that catches your eye is worth a try. Here's a brief list that describes a few different types of potentially enjoyable activities. As you read through this list, see if any of them catch your interest.

- Activities that involve interacting with other people (for example, chatting with the person who helps you in a coffee bar, texting a family member, going out with a friend)

- Activities that involve physical activity (for example, going on a short walk, taking an online yoga class, going to the gym)

- Activities that involve enjoying the outdoors (for example, sitting outside on a park bench, noticing the flowers when you go for a walk, fishing, bicycling, throwing a football around)

- Activities that involve spending time with animals (for example, taking a dog for a walk, playing with a cat, noticing different birds in a park)

- Activities that involve artistic creativity (for example, cooking a new recipe, decorating your home, drawing, singing, playing the guitar)

- Activities that involve experiencing physical pleasure (for example, eating or drinking food you really like, taking a bath, going to a spa, sitting in the sun)

- Activities that involve doing things for yourself (for example, listening to music, reading a favorite book, doing crossword puzzles)

We've posted a much longer, more detailed list called *Ideas for Enjoyable Activities* online. Take some time to read through this list—it can actually be kind of fun. Some of the activities may really resonate with you, others not so much. But we think you may start to get some good ideas!

Maya was initially skeptical about how useful it would be to look at a list of enjoyable activities, but she decided to try. When she looked over the list, two things immediately jumped out for her. First, when she was at college she loved spending hours with her drawing pad, so she wondered if sketching was something she might like again. She laughed when she mentioned the second activity. She had never been to a spa and wondered if it might be fun.

What About You?

Now that you've had the chance to review a list of enjoyable activities, let's see if you can choose a few that you may want to add to your life. Start by choosing two or three activities from the list that you think you might enjoy or that you would have enjoyed before you were depressed. Even if you think you would enjoy them only a little bit, that's okay!

1. _____
2. _____
3. _____

A Quick Review

We've now looked at three strategies for identifying your pleasurable mood-boosting behaviors: building on what's already working; doing what you used to enjoy; and using a list to get ideas for activities you might enjoy. You used each of these strategies to identify two or three activities that you might want to incorporate into your life. Now look over those activities and narrow them down to two or three that you would be most willing to try in the coming week.

1. _____
2. _____
3. _____

We'll come back to these activities in just a moment. First, we want to help you develop an effective plan.

How to Make an Effective Plan

It's now time to make a plan for engaging in the pleasurable mood-boosting activities that you'd like to try. We're going to consider five key components of an effective behavioral activation plan. These components are really important—the more your plan includes all five of them, the more likely it is that you'll follow through on your plan.

Is My Plan Specific?

Often our plans are vague or overly general—more like wishful thinking. Plans such as *This week I'm going to clean up my desk*, or *Someday I'll go on a diet*, or *I'll take my car in for an oil change soon* are really more like good intentions, rather than real plans. Effective plans, by contrast, are specific.

A specific plan answers these five questions:

What will you do?

Who, if anyone, will you do it with?

When will you do it?

Where will you do it?

For how long will you do it?

Let's look at an example. Maya wanted to play board games with her children. This was a vague plan, so she tried to make it more specific. Maya decided that she would let her children choose a game (what), and that she would play with them (who) in the family room (where) for a half hour (how long) on Monday and Thursday at 7:00 p.m. right after dinner (when). When Maya made her plan more specific, it felt easier for her to carry through with it.

Is My Plan Doable?

Once you have a specific plan, it's time to look at whether that plan is doable. You want to be sure you have everything you need to start your plan. A client of Nina's wanted to start running again—she had to find her running shoes in the back of her closet. You also want to be sure that the activities you choose are realistic given your present mood and physical condition. When we're depressed, activities that were easy in the past can be hard to do—even enjoyable ones!

Try to rate each activity that you want to add to your life in terms of how doable it feels. A "1" means that the activity feels very easy to do, and a "10" means that the activity feels very difficult—maybe even impossible—to do.

Ed listed several activities he thought he might want to try this coming week. He liked the idea of getting his old life back, but it also felt hopeless, and he wasn't sure where to start.

Ed first looked at whether these activities were still possible given his injury, and if he had to modify them in some way. He then rated each activity in terms of how doable it felt. He considered whether he had everything he needed to do the activity and also how doable it felt emotionally. Here are Ed's activities and ratings.

Activity	How doable is this activity? 1 (very easy) to 10 (very difficult)
Walking with my wife	3
Going out for dinner with my wife	4
Having family or friends over for a barbecue	5
Seeing my old hockey buddies	8

When Ed looked over his ratings, he decided that he could start walking with his wife, and that he and his wife could go out for dinner. He also thought having some friends or family over for a barbecue might be possible. Seeing his old hockey buddies seemed too hard right now. Rating how doable these activities were gave Ed a sense of hope and provided an idea of where to start.

Take a moment and think about the pleasurable mood-boosting activities you have identified for yourself. Then, use the space below to list the activities and then give them a rating based on how doable they feel right now. Ask yourself, *Do I have everything I need to start the activity?* and *Are these activities realistic for me given my current state of mind, or am I aiming too high?* It's much better to start small.

Activity	How doable is this activity? 1 (very easy) to 10 (very difficult)

What was it like to ask yourself how doable the activity felt? How could you make these activities even more doable? Would it help to scale down the activities you identified even a little? Write down your thoughts here:

_____

_____

_____

_____

_____

_____

_____

Now it's time for you to write down your plan. Be sure to keep it somewhere that you can easily see.

What About You?

Let's check if your mood-boosting activities are specific. First, write down those two or three mood-boosting activities you would like to add to your life this coming week. Then try to complete the *Developing Effective Plans* worksheet on the next page.

Were your mood-boosting activities specific? If yes, great! If not, think about how you could make them more specific. Did completing the *Developing Effective Plans* worksheet change how doable the activities felt?

Developing Effective Plans

What am I going to do?	Who will I do it with?	When will I do it?	Where will I do it?	How long will I do it for?	Is it doable?
1.					
2.					
3.					

Can I Make This Activity Part of My Routine?

Establishing a good routine—one that includes engaging in enjoyable and meaningful activities on a regular basis—is the foundation of a good, depression-resistant life. Special activities such as joyful holidays are really just the icing on the cake. If the cake underneath is dry and unappetizing, you won't want to eat it despite the delicious icing. If you are depressed, having a good routine is especially important. Special treats are great—but it's having a life of daily mood-boosting activities that is more likely to help lift you out of your depression and create a better life.

Take a moment to reflect on the activities you identified earlier. Are they activities that can become part of your regular routine? How could you make them a regular part of your life? Write down your thoughts here:

_____

_____

_____

_____

_____

_____

Have I Targeted the Lowest Part of My Day?

We all have periods of the day when our mood tends to be at its lowest. Look over your *Daily Activities* worksheet to see your lowest time of the day. It's important to make sure that when you plan your mood-boosting activities, some of them target this time period.

Let's take the case of Taylor, another one of Nina's clients, as an example. Taylor tended to stay in bed for an hour in the morning thinking about how hard their life was. Their mood would get worse and worse and by the time they got up they didn't feel like doing anything. Nina and Taylor worked out a plan where Taylor would set the alarm for 8:30 a.m. and then get right out of bed as soon as it went off—even if they didn't feel like it. They put on some music and had a cup of tea and toast with their favorite jam. When the alarm went off they would tell themselves they had toast and jam waiting. They found it helpful to have something pleasant in their morning routine to look forward to—even if it was just toast and jam.

Taylor's plan was doable, specific, and could easily become part of a routine. As a bonus, it targeted the very time of the day that Taylor's mood was at its lowest.

What is the lowest part of your day?

_____

What is one thing you can build into that part of your day that you can look forward to?

_____

Have I Planned for Obstacles?

An effective plan involves identifying the possible obstacles that can pop up and get in the way of a behavioral activation plan. While we can't possibly identify *every* obstacle, it's helpful to flag as many as possible. One way to do this is to close your eyes and imagine yourself engaging in one of your mood-boosting activities. As vividly as possible, visualize every step of the activity. Then note what could get in the way of your plan. Here are some questions that can help identify your obstacles:

- Is the activity too hard or too complex; do I need to scale it down?

- Are there some real-life obstacles that could get in the way?

- Might I forget to follow my behavioral activation plan ?

- Might I be tempted to give in to my depressed feelings of not wanting to do anything rather than following my behavioral activation plan?

Use the *My Obstacles* worksheet to record as many of the potential obstacles for your planned mood-boosting activity as possible. Then, beside each obstacle, come up with possible solutions or ways you could work around the problem.

My Obstacles	
Activity:	
Obstacle	**Possible solution or workaround**

Imaginal Rehearsal

Before you engage in a mood-boosting activity, you may find it helpful to go through it in your imagination. It's a strategy called "imaginal rehearsal." Elite athletes use it routinely to practice their skills and improve their performance (Blankert and Hamstra 2016). We think it can work for you too.

Start by choosing a mood-boosting activity. When you are ready, close your eyes and take a few deep breaths. Now imagine yourself taking the first step toward engaging in the activity you've chosen. Visualize it as vividly and in as much detail as you can. Try to see yourself actually doing the activity, step by step. Imagine yourself enjoying the activity.

Repeat this three times.

What was imaginal rehearsal like for you? Did your experience of the activity change as you repeated the image? Jot down your observations in the space below.

_____

_____

_____

Research has found that mentally rehearsing an activity increases your chance of doing it successfully (Hays 2012). Try making imaginal rehearsal a regular habit as you try more of the various mood-boosting activities that we discuss throughout this workbook.

Take the Plunge!

At this point you've made a specific plan to engage in a pleasurable mood-boosting activity. Now it's time to put your plan into action—to take the plunge—and then see how it goes.

One way to evaluate how well your behavioral activation plan is working is to rate your mood both before and after engaging in your chosen activity. The *Rate My Mood* worksheet is an easy way to do this. Try to get into the habit of using this worksheet each time you implement a behavioral activation plan. We suggest you make a few copies of it—we'll be using them frequently throughout the rest of this workbook. Although we've left space for three activities, as you go through the book you may have fewer or more activities you want to rate.

Rate My Mood			
Activity	Date of activity	Mood before activity 1 (very depressed) to 10 (very happy)	Mood after activity 1 (very depressed) to 10 (very happy)

What's Next?

In this chapter you started developing your own list of mood-boosting activities that you personally enjoy and that bring you pleasure. You also made an effective plan to take action on one or two of them in the coming week. This illustration summarizes the strategies we used to identify your mood-boosting activities.

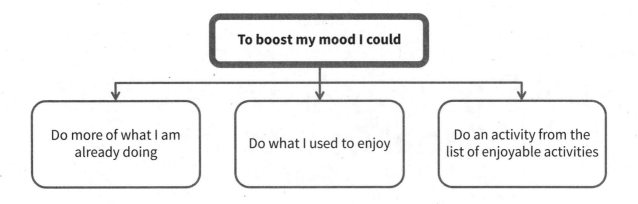

Figure 3.1: Pleasurable Mood-Boosting Activities

Take a moment to reflect on what resonated most strongly with you as you read this chapter. What can you take with you into your life?

_____

_____

What steps can you plan to take in the coming week?

_____

_____

What can you do to ensure that your behavioral activation plan will be successful?

_____

_____

In the next chapter we're going to look at what research tells us about two additional building blocks of a depression-resistant life: physical exercise and social connections. We're going to look at how you can incorporate these two important activities into your behavioral activation plan.

CHAPTER 4

Get Physically Active and Make Social Connections

Physical activity and social connections are two of the activities that are most likely to boost your mood and reset the depressed brain's bias toward negativity. However, depression being what it is, physical activity and social connections are precisely the kinds of activities that tend to get dropped when we're feeling down. Let's see how you can improve your mood by adding these activities to your life—step by step.

Engage in Regular Physical Activity

The research is clear: physical exercise is good for your mental health (Chekroud et al. 2018), and people who engage in regular physical exercise are less likely to become depressed (Pearce et al. 2022). If you are already depressed, physical exercise can be an effective treatment for your depression. Studies have shown that depressed patients who are prescribed a course of physical exercise for their depression improve just as much as patients treated with antidepressant medication (Josefsson, Lindwall, and Archer 2014). The evidence suggests that a brisk walk will help your mood more than a slow stroll, but any movement is good. Over time, people who continue to exercise have a lower likelihood of slipping back into depression (Blumenthal et al. 2007; Chekroud et al. 2018).

Almost any kind of physical activity can improve your mood. It doesn't have to be a vigorous workout. Let's try a thought experiment. Think about a time when you went for a walk or did some exercise when you were feeling down or after a stressful day. First, write down what you did.

_____

Then think about these questions, and write down your thoughts.

What happened to your mood after the walk or exercise?

_____

If you noticed any additional benefits, write them down.

_____

_____

What did you learn from this thought experiment?

_____

_____

_____

How Does Physical Activity Boost Your Mood?

Regular physical activity has a direct impact on our brain chemistry, which, in turn, affects our mood. To give you some examples, when we exercise we increase the neurotransmitters serotonin and dopamine in our brains (Lin and Kuo 2013); we reduce the levels of cortisol, a hormone associated with stress and low mood (Beserra et al. 2018); and we increase the levels of neurochemicals responsible for the growth and development of new brain tissue (Miranda et al. 2019; Basso and Suzuki 2017). Although the exact mechanisms of change aren't completely clear, we know for sure that regular exercise changes our brains in ways that have a positive impact on our mood.

Exercise also affects our psychology. For example, exercising can improve your sleep and may affect how you feel about yourself. When we move more and we feel better in our bodies, we also feel more self-confident. For many people, exercising can provide a real sense of accomplishment.

One more point: there is good evidence that physical activity done outdoors in nature can boost your mood even more than when it's done indoors (Barton and Pretty 2010). This makes total sense to us. I (Nina) am far happier walking outside than walking on a treadmill inside my somewhat dark condo gym—add a friend and a stop for a cappuccino, and I start to feel quite cheerful!

How to Incorporate Physical Activity into Your Life

With so many benefits, you'd think that it would be a no-brainer (so to speak) that we'd all be out there happily walking, running, pumping iron, and moving in whatever way we can. The reality, however, is that only about a quarter of us exercise regularly (Abildso et al. 2023). And when we're depressed—feeling tired, lacking in energy and motivation—the idea of moving at all feels even more overwhelming.

So how can we get moving? We're going to follow the same approach we took in chapter 3. First, we'll help you choose a mood-boosting physical activity that works for you, and then we'll help you come up with a specific plan for incorporating it into your life.

The first step is to choose an activity. We are going to suggest three strategies you can use to find a physical activity that works for you.

Grow what you are already doing or get back to what you used to do. Any increase in physical activity is a huge accomplishment, and it will begin to boost your mood. You can start by noticing what you are already doing and then try to increase it just a bit. It can also be helpful to identify physical activities that you used to enjoy but have stopped doing.

Start with something really, really simple. What about a five-minute walk a few times per week? Or, if you are already walking, maybe walk a little longer or a little faster? Maybe you could stretch in the morning—or if you're already stretching, maybe you could attend a yoga class or even a workout in the gym with a friend. Remember, *anything* is better than nothing!

What is one physical activity you are already doing that you could increase?

_____

Is there something you used to enjoy that you could add to your life?

_____

Get physical activity from things you enjoy. Try to think of a physical activity you enjoy. It could be a simple activity, such as a walk around the block, or a more vigorous walk with a friend. Some people like to swim or participate in games or sports; for example, soccer, tennis, golf, baseball, pickleball. Anything is good. One of Nina's clients loved to dance, so she decided to dance to a music video in her living room. She had fun. Even a small change is good!

What is one physical activity you enjoy that you could add to your life? Write it down here:

_____

Integrate physical activity into your everyday life. You can get a really good mood boost by adding small amounts of activity to your regular life. For example, rather than driving to work, could you walk or cycle instead? Maybe you could try parking a little farther away than usual so that you have to walk a bit more? Perhaps you could do some stretching while watching TV, or take a walk on your lunch break. Housework can also be a good way to add physical activity—you bend, lift, and push when vacuuming. We're sure you can think of many ways of "sneaking" more physical activity into your everyday life.

Try to make your physical activities more enjoyable. Can you think of ways to get some enjoyment from everyday activities that require physical effort? I (Nina) live a fifteen-minute walk from the subway. I discovered a podcast I like to listen to as I walk. It's made what was a boring walk into something I look forward to. A friend of mine listens to great music while vacuuming. While working in the garden, a client of Stephen's talks on their smartphone to their best friend, who lives in another city.

How can you make your everyday life more physically active? Think of small changes—they really add up—and write them here.

_____

_____

_____

How can you get more enjoyment from physical activities or chores that you have to engage in anyway?

_____

_____

_____

_____

Develop an Action Plan

Now that you've identified a few steps you could take to increase your physical activity, it's time to make a plan and take action. Try to identify the first step in your plan. Be sure that this step is specific and doable, and could be part of your routine. Finally, be sure to identify and problem solve any obstacles you might encounter.

Below, you'll find an *Action Plan* worksheet that you can use to incorporate these activities into your daily life. We've included an item from Ed's action plan as an example.

Action Plan: Physical Activity

What I'll do	Is my plan...	My first step	Obstacles I may encounter	How I'll handle these obstacles
Walk Alex to daycare at 8:00 on Tuesdays and Thursdays; walk back home	☑ specific? ☑ doable? ☑ part of my routine?	Talk to my wife to learn what Alex needs for daycare, so I can pack his knapsack.	It may be hard to get up in the morning.	Set alarm, remember I promised Alex and my wife I would take him to daycare
	☐ specific? ☐ doable? ☐ part of my routine?			
	☐ specific? ☐ doable? ☐ part of my routine?			
	☐ specific? ☐ doable? ☐ part of my routine?			

Take a moment to reflect on what was it like to make a plan and write it down. Could any of these activities target the lowest part of your day?

It can be helpful to monitor how much you exercise. For the more technologically inclined, smartwatches and fitness trackers can provide feedback regarding your levels of activity. You can then use this feedback to slowly increase your activity. As a bonus, smart devices can also provide you with gentle reminders to stay physically active. For example, I (Nina) tend to think I do a lot more exercise than I actually do. I'm always sure my phone underestimates my steps! You can also monitor your physical activity on the *Daily Activities* worksheet or any other monitoring system.

Cultivate Social Connections

Human beings are social creatures. Scores of research studies have shown that our happiness and well-being are closely linked to our social relationships (Diener and Seligman 2002). One Harvard study followed a group of 724 people from the time they were teenagers in 1938. The study found that having positive social relationships was the strongest predictor of health and happiness (Waldinger and Schulz 2023). On the flip side, we also know that loneliness is closely related to depression (Cacioppo et al. 2006). People differ in how many and what type of relationships they need, but everyone needs some social connections.

As we saw in chapter 1, depression makes us want to withdraw and distance ourselves from others. Over time, we become lonely and even more depressed. However, connecting with other people is a powerful mood-boosting strategy that can counteract loneliness and depression. This is why we consider activities that involve connecting with others to be the third building block of a happy, fulfilling, depression-resistant life.

How to Connect with Others

When you're feeling depressed, the prospect of interacting with others may feel overwhelming. Your mind will probably give you all sorts of reasons to avoid social interaction; for example, *People will dislike me; I'll feel worse; I'll have nothing to say; I don't have the energy.* It can be hard to know how to get started.

Below are a few steps you can take to increase your social interactions and begin feeling better. As we go through each of these strategies, take a moment to see how they could apply to you.

See More of the People You're Already Seeing

You want to grow your connections with people who boost your mood. Think of people who are already in your life. Is there a friend, a neighbor, a colleague, or a person at the grocery store that you enjoy talking to sometimes? Are there people in your life who are experiencing the same problem as you? Would it feel helpful to talk to them more often? This might be another parent home with a toddler, another new person at your place of work, or someone else who just moved into the neighborhood. Take a moment to brainstorm people you could connect with. Write their names here:

_____

_____

Could you see them more often and maybe for longer periods of time? I (Nina) was in the middle of writing this section when I went to get a cappuccino (I know, I probably drink too much coffee). My barista started talking about a sporting event she had seen on TV that I had also watched. We chatted for a couple of minutes—I left with a smile.

Reach Out

Can you think of someone you haven't seen for a while, someone you might enjoy connecting with again? It might be an old friend or acquaintance, a family member, a work colleague, or a neighbor. What about someone you don't know well but who has something in common with you? Who is someone you could reach out to? Write down their name here:

_____

Start with something really simple. What about sending a short text message or email just to say hello? How could you reach out to the person you identified? Jot down your ideas here:

_____

_____

You might be surprised at how happy people are to hear from you—even if you've been out of touch for a while!

Meet Up, Join Up

If you want to meet new people, think about whether you cross paths with anyone you might like to get to know, perhaps someone you see on the train or the bus every day, or someone you see at school or work. Could you start slowly and say hello?

You might also consider looking for a group to join—a sports league, a class, a parents' group, a book club, a religious congregation, or an organization that corresponds to your interests. Many community centers offer support groups that can help if you are facing a particular difficult situation. If meeting in person seems a bit too daunting, consider joining an online community. Interacting with others online can be supportive and rewarding. In-person meetups are probably the gold standard, but connecting online is a great way to start.

Ask yourself, *Is there someone in my life I would like to get to know better?* Write down their name.

_____

Is there an organization of people with similar interests or experiences that I could join? Write down its name.

_____

What specific steps could you take to connect to this person or join this organization?

_____

_____

_____

Help Out

Helping others can be a big mood booster. You may have a friend, a neighbor, or a family member who could use a helping hand. Volunteering is a great way to connect with people who may share some of your values and interests. Many food banks, local hospitals, animal shelters, religious organizations, and other community agencies have websites posting available volunteer positions. That's often a good place to start. Ask yourself, *Is there someone in my life I could help out, or an organization that could use a volunteer?* Write down the name of person or organization.

_____

Be Friendly

Stephen's wife once tried an experiment. She smiled at people wherever she went. She was amazed at the results. Not only did smiling brighten her own mood, but people were friendly back to her. There is good research evidence that smiling and saying hello, even to people you don't know, such as the person who helps you with your groceries at the checkout counter, can boost your mood (Vrugt and Vet 2009). If you've been alone in your home, getting out, smiling, and saying hello to almost anyone is a good first step.

How could you be a little more friendly this week? Who is someone you could smile at? Write down your ideas in the space below.

_____

_____

_____

Maya liked the first strategy—increasing contact with people she was already seeing. Last week she walked with her colleague Rava at lunchtime and was surprised at how much she enjoyed it. She wondered if Rava was interested in regularly walking with her. Maya also liked the idea of trying to smile more at people when she was out.

What About You?

Take a look at all the ideas you came up with for adding enjoyable social interactions to your life. Identify one or two that you would like to try this coming week. Next, make a specific, doable plan that can be part of your routine. Remember, we also want you to identify the first step in making the plan happen, and then plan for that first step. Don't forget to identify and problem solve any obstacles. Try to complete the *Action Plan: Social Connections* worksheet. We included Maya's plan as an example.

Action Plan: Social Connections				
What I'll do	Is my plan...	My first step	Obstacles I may encounter	How I'll handle these obstacles
Walk with Rava for 30 minutes every day at lunchtime	☑ specific? ☑ doable? ☑ part of my routine?	Text Rava tonight after the kids are asleep	I may be anxious	I will tell myself to just do it, and that I have a plan
Smile at more people, starting with the cashier in the grocery store at checkout on Tuesday	☑ specific? ☑ doable? ☑ part of my routine?	Go to the grocery store	Feeling silly	Use imaginal rehearsal to practice in my imagination
	☐ specific? ☐ doable? ☐ part of my routine?			
	☐ specific? ☐ doable? ☐ part of my routine?			

If at First You Don't Succeed…

It can be *really* hard to start incorporating more physical exercise and more social activity into your life, especially when you're feeling depressed. So, if at first you don't manage to do it, please be kind and compassionate to yourself. Recognize that this is hard. It might help to use imaginal rehearsal to visualize yourself succeeding. You may also find it helpful to circle back to the *My Obstacles* worksheet at the end of chapter 3. Use the worksheet to identify and plan for any previously unforeseen obstacles. Don't give up. It may take a few tries. Once you start, we think being physically active and making a few more social connections will make a real difference in your mood.

What's Next?

We've started creating a solid behavioral activation plan that will help you push back on your depression and improve your mood. So far we've looked at three building block activities—activities that you find enjoyable (that is, pleasurable mood-boosting activities) in chapter 3, and physical exercise and social connections in this chapter. This illustration provides a good summary of what we've covered.

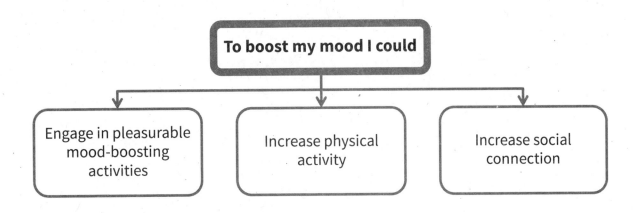

Figure 4.1: Effective Mood-Boosting Behavior: Physical Activity and Social Connection

As you reflect on this chapter, what was the most important takeaway for you?

_____

_____

How do you plan to apply what you learned to your daily life?

_____

_____

_____

_____

_____

In the next chapter, we're going to help you supercharge the effectiveness of your behavior activation plans by identifying activities that align with your personal values. So let's get personal!

CHAPTER 5

Don't Forget Your Values— They're Important!

Adding mood-boosting activities into our lives—pleasurable activities, physical exercise, and social interaction—is an important step in overcoming depression and feeling better—but it's not the whole story. Creating a truly good life also involves engaging in activities that give us a sense of meaning and purpose—activities that reflect our own unique personal values. Research has clearly shown that when behavioral activation includes activities that are consistent with our values it is even more effective in combating depression (Kanter et al. 2010). That's why values-based activities represent the fourth building block to a good depression-resistant life.

What Are Values?

Simply put, our values are whatever we truly consider to be most important in our lives. Values can take the form of personal qualities or attributes that we admire and see as being central to who we are or what we most want to be (for example, honesty, curiosity, adventurousness, generosity, fairness). Values can also reflect ideals (for example, family, friendship, physical fitness, freedom, wealth, simplicity, spirituality) that we cherish, aspire to, and see as critical elements of a good, satisfying life.

Values play a big role in our lives. They help us make decisions and guide our actions. When we act in ways that are at odds with our values, we experience an uncomfortable sense of dissonance, discomfort, and dissatisfaction. On the other hand, when our behavior aligns with our values, life is more meaningful and we experience a powerful boost to our mood and a sense of purpose.

Identify Your Values

The first step toward incorporating values-based activities into your life is to clearly identify your values. Because our values are so deeply rooted, it's not always that easy to identify them off the top of our heads. If you were asked "What are your values?" it wouldn't be surprising if you drew a blank. When we're depressed, it's particularly difficult to spontaneously describe our values—we often feel that nothing is all that important or meaningful.

Look at a List

One way to identify your values is to look at a list of commonly held values and choose about ten of them that you feel are the most important to you. Take a few minutes to read through the values listed here. It's by no means an exhaustive list—there are literally hundreds and hundreds of values. We've also left lots of room for you to add your own.

Table 5.1: List of Values

Rate how important each value is to you on a 5-point scale where 1 = not very important and 5 = very important.

Achievement	_____	**Creativity**	_____
Growth	_____	Adventure	_____
Status	_____	Curiosity	_____
Success	_____	Exploration	_____
Wealth	_____	Imagination	_____
		Originality	_____

Knowledge _____

Intelligence _____

Learning _____

Wisdom _____

Good feelings _____

Compassion _____

Contentment _____

Gratitude _____

Happiness _____

Kindness _____

Love _____

Order _____

Certainty _____

Conformity _____

Control _____

Punctuality _____

Security _____

Health _____

Energy _____

Fitness _____

Mental health _____

Social connections _____

Cooperation _____

Equality _____

Family _____

Forgiveness _____

Friendship _____

Kindness _____

Generosity _____

Loyalty _____

Selflessness _____

Service _____

Tolerance _____

Spirituality _____

Beauty _____

Devotion _____

Faith _____

Forgiveness _____

Humility _____

Meaning _____

Peacefulness _____

Simplicity _____

Personal strength _____

Ambition _____

Assertiveness _____

Confidence _____

Courage _____

Dedication _____

Discipline _____

Self-reliance _____

Toughness _____

Enjoyment _____

Fun _____

Excitement _____

Humor _____

Playfulness _____

Spontaneity _____

Surprise _____

Independence _____

Freedom _____

Individuality _____

Competence _____

Efficiency _____

Hard work _____

Leadership _____

Professionalism _____

Integrity _____

Authenticity _____

Dependability _____

Fairness _____

Honesty _____

Reputation _____

Responsibility _____

Self-respect _____

Sincerity _____

Trustworthiness _____

Other values

_____ _____

_____ _____

_____ _____

_____ _____

_____ _____

_____ _____

Place a checkmark beside the ten values that are most important to you. Next, we're going to ask you some very personal questions to help you identify your values even more clearly and specifically.

What Are Your Happiest Experiences?

Thinking back to the times in our lives when we were the happiest can provide helpful insights into our values—especially if we reflect on *why* these experiences made us so happy. For example, when I (Stephen) asked Ed about his happiest experiences, Ed remembered the day he proposed to his wife (and she accepted!). Ed looked at the list of values he checked as most important. He then picked the values that he felt were associated with his happiness on that day. He chose "family" and "love."

Try to identify the values associated with your happiest moments. First, list three of the happiest moments of your life; then reflect on why you felt so happy on each occasion. Next, look back at the list of values and for each of these experiences, write down the values you think may have contributed to your happiness.

My happy experience

_____

What values are associated with that experience?

_____

My happy experience

_____

What values are associated with that experience?

_____

My happy experience

_____

What values are associated with that experience?

_____

When we're very depressed, it can be difficult to recall happy experiences in our lives. If that's the case for you, don't worry. There are several other ways to identify your values.

Who Do You Most Admire?

We tend to admire people who exhibit or represent our most deeply held values. The people we admire could be public figures, family members, or acquaintances. Nina asked Maya to identify three people she really admired. She immediately mentioned the principal at her school. She valued the principal's strong work ethic and fairness. She also admired the singer Taylor Swift for her creativity and for being a groundbreaker. Maya's responses provided us with important clues about her values.

Below, list three people you admire, and then reflect on what it is about those people that makes you think so highly of them. Using the list of values as a reference, see if you can identify the values represented in the lives of these three people.

Person I admire _____

What values does this person represent? _____

Person I admire _____

What values does this person represent? _____

Person I admire _____

What values does this person represent? _____

Who Do You Want to Be?

Think about the kind of person you'd like to be and the kind of life you'd like to have. Try to imagine yourself in the future—say, at your own eightieth birthday party. We're going to ask you two important questions to help you identify your values. Write down your answers below.

What would you like to see as you look back over your life?

_____

_____

_____

_____

What would you like to hear people say about you—the kind of person you were, the things you spent your time on, the qualities you embodied?

_____

_____

_____

Now look at the values you checked as most important. See if you can write down the values that best capture these qualities.

_____

_____

_____

_____

When Ed did this exercise, he initially had some difficulty defining who he wanted to be. It was easier to imagine what he wanted people to say about him on his eightieth birthday. He told Stephen he wanted to be known first and foremost as a good father, a good husband, and a good friend. He also wanted people to respect him for having the courage to deal with his physical problems. He then picked the values of family, friendship, courage, and determination as some of the values arising from this exercise.

Your Core Values

Now that you've had the chance to identify your values in several different ways, let's pull it all together. Looking back over the exercises, create a list of the five to ten values that you think are most important to you. We'll call these your "core values" because they're at the heart of what's really important to you. Try to list them in the order of their priority, starting with the value that is most central. It's okay if you're not clear on the order of your values; you can also just make a list of the ten most important. This is not meant to be a list of all your values—just your ten most important ones.

1. _____

2. _____

3. _____

4. _____

5. _____

6. _____

7. _____

8. _____

9. _____

10. _____

Turn Your Values into Mood-Boosting Activities

Now that you've identified your core values, we're going to ask you to take the next step—translating those values into specific, doable actions that you can incorporate into your life. Values-based activities can really challenge your depression by supercharging the mood-boosting effects of behavioral activation and improving motivation.

Let's start by choosing one of the values you've flagged as most important to you. Next, we'll identify some activities you could engage in that would be consistent with this important value. Make sure that the activities you identify are specific and doable, and can be part of your routine.

Ed really valued family relationships, so we'll use that as an example. He immediately thought of spending more time with Alex as an example of valuing family relationships. This was a really good start and it was doable, but Ed and Stephen agreed that it needed to be more specific. Ed narrowed it down and came up with the idea of taking Alex to the park for an hour on Saturday morning. This was much more specific.

What About You?

Now it's time to bring values-based activities into your life. Choose a value that is important to you. Next, list the value and at least one or two associated behaviors on the *From Values to Actions* worksheet below. We've included Ed's response as an example. You can do this exercise for as many of your core values as you'd like. As always, the key is to make sure that the activities you come up with are specific and doable.

If you're having trouble coming up with ideas, here's a strategy that might help. Imagine that you and a stranger are participants in a game show called "Values Charades." You'll win a million dollars if the other person can guess your most important values. You're not allowed to talk to the other person—they only get to watch what you do over a one-week period. What activities would you engage in to help them guess your core values? Those are a good start to identifying your values-based activities.

From Values to Action	
Core value	**Specific and doable values-based activities**
Family relationships	Spending more time with Alex–taking him to the park on Saturday morning Spending quality time with my wife–no screens during dinner

Let's Make a Plan

At the gym where Stephen goes to exercise there's a motivational slogan written in huge black letters on the entrance wall. We like it. It says, "What is *one* thing I can do today that will get me a little bit closer to where I want to be (or who I want to be) tomorrow?" In other words, what activity can I engage in today that will be consistent with the important values in my life?

Take a look at what activities you came up with when you completed the *From Values to Actions* worksheet. Now pick one or two of these activities to schedule into your life using the *Action Plan: Values-Based Activities* worksheet. Write down when and where you will do the activity and how long it will take. In addition, check that the activity is specific and doable, and can be part of your routine. Finally, record the first step you'll need to take, and reflect on any obstacles you may encounter. We've included one of Ed's responses as an example.

Action Plan: Values-Based Activities

What I'll do	What value will this honor?	Is my plan...	My first step	Obstacles I may encounter	How I'll handle these obstacles
Take Alex to the park for one hour on Saturday mornings	Family relationships	☑ specific? ☑ doable? ☑ part of my routine?	Alex and I will get dressed for the weather	Rainy weather	We'll go to an indoor play space instead.
		☐ specific? ☐ doable? ☐ part of my routine?			
		☐ specific? ☐ doable? ☐ part of my routine?			
		☐ specific? ☐ doable? ☐ part of my routine?			

Do you remember imaginal rehearsal from chapter 3? Now is a good time to use it. Close your eyes and take a deep breath, then imagine doing the activity you chose. In as much detail as possible feel yourself taking the first step. Then imagine doing the whole activity. Allow yourself to feel good that you are doing an activity that is consistent with your values. Repeat the imagery exercise three times. What was that like for you? Did it start to feel more doable?

Now, it's time to put your plan into action! As you've done earlier, be sure to record your mood before and after engaging in these activities. You can use the *Rate My Mood* worksheet that we introduced in the previous chapter. We're confident that as you do this—step by step and day by day—you will discover why values-based activities are such powerful mood-boosting behaviors.

Supercharge Your Mood-Boosting Activities with Values

In chapters 3 and 4 we introduced you to a number of activities that can boost your mood. We'll be adding a few more types of mood-boosting activities in the next couple of chapters. You can make these activities even more powerful if you identify ways in which they are not just mood-boosting but also meaningful. When we do activities that are both mood-boosting and related to our values there is extra potential for boosting both our mood *and* our motivation.

In the illustration below, we have listed some possible mood-boosting activities and their related core values. You will see that some activities are related mostly to one core value and some are related to more than one value.

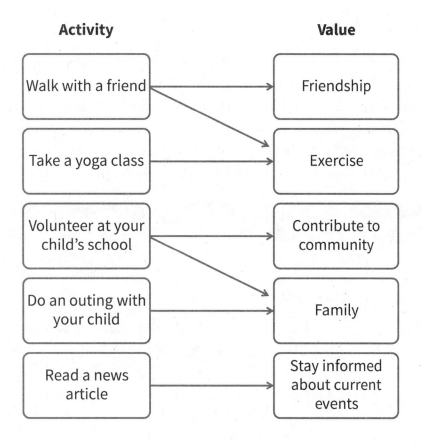

Figure 5.1: Mood-Boosting Activities and Their Related Values

One of the mood-boosting activities Maya wanted to include in her week was playing board games with her children. As her week progressed, she found it hard to get motivated. There was always something else that seemed more pressing. Maya wondered if identifying her core values related to playing board games with her children might increase her motivation. She looked at her list of core values and realized that playing board games with her children was related to the values of being a good mother and a mother who did fun things with her children. Identifying her values did not always make it easy to find the time and motivation to play, but it increased her commitment and motivation. She also took additional pleasure and a sense of accomplishment from the activity.

What About You?

Using the *Supercharge My Mood-Boosting Activities with My Values* worksheet, list two or three of the activities from chapter 3 or 4 that you identified as mood boosters. Now, take a moment to think about why they are important to you. How are they related to any of your core values? For example, if you identified going for a walk with a friend as a mood-boosting activity, is this related to the value of being fit, the value of being in nature, or maybe the value of friendship? It could be that all of these values are important to you. We've included Maya's response as an example.

Supercharge My Mood-Boosting Activities with My Values	
Mood-boosting activity	**Related value**
Maya: Playing board games with my children	Being a good mother Being a mother who does fun activities with her children
1.	
2.	
3.	

Let's take a moment to reflect on the exercise you just did. What was it like to identify the values behind your activities? How did it affect your motivation? How did it impact your feelings about completing the activities? Write down your thoughts below.

_____

_____

_____

_____

_____

_____

As you develop action plans for the various mood-boosting activities you choose to incorporate into your life, remember to reflect on the values they represent for you. Why are these activities important to you? How do they move you closer to where—and who—you want to be in the future? Asking yourself these questions will help increase your motivation for your behavioral activation plans and may also increase their mood-boosting potential.

What's Next?

In this chapter, we've gotten a little more personal by exploring what is most important to you—your values. When you think over what we have covered in this chapter, what was important to you? What would help you have a better life and push back on your depression?

_____

_____

How would you like to take what you learned into your daily life?

_____

_____

We've now covered four types of activities that constitute the building blocks of a happy, meaningful, depression-resistant life: (1) pleasurable mood-boosting activities; (2) physical exercise; (3) social connections; and (4) values-based activities. The illustration below provides a summary.

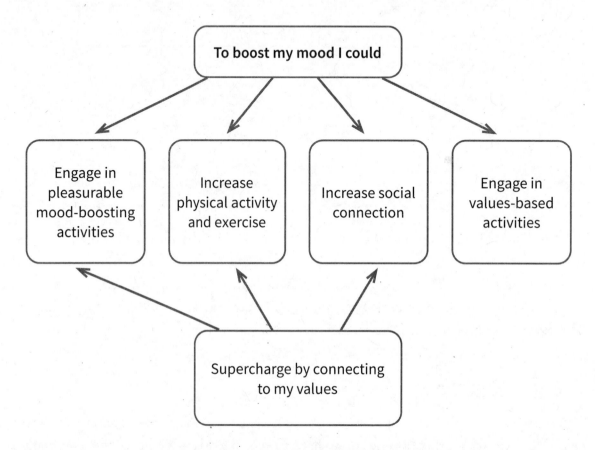

Figure 5.2: Effective Mood-Boosting Behavior: Values-Based Activities

In the next chapter, we're going to focus on another building block that can play an important role in combating depression by not only boosting your mood but also by increasing your sense of self-confidence. We're going to look at activities that promote a sense of mastery and accomplishment.

CHAPTER 6

Create a Sense of Mastery and Accomplishment

Do you remember when you first learned to ride a bicycle? It took a lot of practice—and probably involved a few falls along the way—but eventually you got it. Can you recall the feelings of satisfaction that your success gave you? Perhaps you can think of other similar experiences—the first time you read a chapter book, or when you finally learned to swim or passed your driving test? These are all examples of activities that likely created positive feelings of mastery and accomplishment.

Throughout the course of our lives we continue to have new experiences of mastery and accomplishment—discovering how to use a new smartphone app; learning a new language, game, or sport; graduating from high school or college; getting your first job or a promotion. You can probably think of many others. All these activities involve setting a goal, and then, through sustained effort and persistence, acquiring new skills and knowledge and achieving a level of success.

Even doing everyday tasks can create satisfying feelings of mastery and accomplishment—things like getting to work on time, fixing something around the house, making your bed, cleaning a dirty sink, paying a bill, chopping firewood, or mowing the lawn. Especially when we are depressed, these seemingly everyday activities can represent very significant achievements.

Over time, as we have more and more of these experiences of mastery and accomplishment, we begin to develop what psychologists call "self-efficacy" (Bandura 2008). Self-efficacy is the belief in our own ability to succeed despite obstacles. Increased self-efficacy allows us to face life's challenges with greater calm, resilience, and persistence, because we believe that our efforts will pay off in the end. In addition to building self-efficacy, activities that provide us with a feeling of mastery and accomplishment can contribute to a sense of positive self-esteem. Taken together, they represent very important components of a happy, fulfilling life.

How Does Depression Affect Mastery and Accomplishment?

It probably won't come as too much of a surprise to you to learn that depression actively discourages us from engaging in activities that provide a sense of mastery and accomplishment. Depression makes us feel pessimistic about our ability to achieve our goals, cynical about the value of our accomplishments, and lacking in motivation. We stop taking on new challenges that could provide us with an empowering sense of self-efficacy and stop engaging in activities that could lead to satisfying feelings of achievement. We are left feeling even more empty and depressed. The illustration below shows how this negative cycle works.

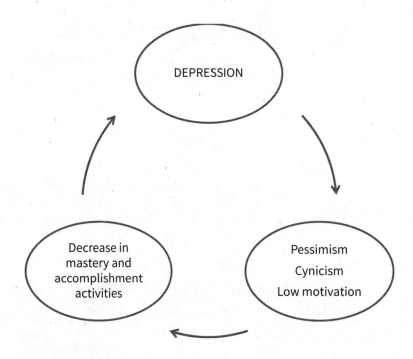

Figure 6.1: The Vicious Cycle of Depression and Mastery/Accomplishment Activities

Prior to becoming depressed, Ed was involved in a number of activities that gave him a sense of mastery and accomplishment. First, Ed was very proud of his work as a carpenter. He wistfully recalled feeling a great sense of satisfaction when he completed his certificate of qualification. Even after qualifying, Ed continued to take additional courses. He hoped to be promoted. When he had to stop working because of his hand pain, Ed lost this important source of personal gratification, and the loss contributed to his depression.

Before his hand injury, Ed used to make small pieces of furniture in his free time. He felt really good about the skill he was developing in this area. After he became depressed, Ed lost interest in making furniture. Instead of spending a few hours in the evening working on small pieces of furniture, Ed watched TV and drank beer. He became even more depressed.

Ed also lost interest in other activities that had previously given him satisfying feelings of accomplishment. For example, prior to his depression, Ed loved taking care of his car. He washed it faithfully every Saturday morning—inside and out—until it gleamed. After becoming depressed, Ed stopped washing his car. As a result, his car often looked a bit shabby. Ed didn't want to be seen driving a dirty car, so he stayed home and felt even worse.

What About You?

Let's see if you've disengaged from activities that give you a sense of mastery and accomplishment. Think back to some of the things you did in the past that gave you a satisfying sense of achievement and success. You can list these in the first column of the *My Previous Mastery and Accomplishment Activities* worksheet below. Include both "big" mastery and accomplishment activities as well as your more everyday achievements. In the second column, note how frequently you engaged in those activities in the past. In the third column, rate how frequently you engage in this activity now. We've included Ed's responses as examples.

My Previous Mastery and Accomplishment Activities		
Previous mastery and accomplishment activities	Frequency before I became depressed	Frequency now
Completing my carpentry apprenticeship	Completed 3 years ago	n/a
Washing my car	Weekly	Once or twice a year
Working on my small furniture projects	2-3 times per week	Never

Previous mastery and accomplishment activities	Frequency before I became depressed	Frequency now

Take a moment to reflect on what you learned from completing this worksheet. What change did you notice in how often you're engaging in your previous mastery and accomplishment activities?

_____

_____

_____

Which activities—if any—have changed, and how has this impacted your mood?

_____

_____

_____

To what degree has depression stopped you from taking on new challenges and from engaging in activities that gave you a satisfying sense of self-efficacy and self-esteem?

_____

_____

_____

What activities related to a sense of mastery or accomplishment have you stopped engaging in because of your feelings of depression?

_____

_____

_____

How has this impacted your mood?

_____

_____

_____

The encouraging news is that you can push back and recapture your sense of mastery and accomplishment. We're going to show you how.

Identify Your Mastery and Accomplishment Activities

In the next section we're going to give you some strategies for identifying mastery and accomplishment activities that can help you reverse the negative cycle of depression, improve your sense of self-efficacy and self-esteem, and create positive feelings of achievement.

Notice What You're Already Doing

You may be engaging in a number of mastery and accomplishment activities already, but either not noticing them or not giving yourself any or enough credit for them. Think about all the things you do—big and small—that require some degree of effort, attention, and persistence. These could be activities that may seem unimportant to you (especially when you're feeling depressed), but that contribute to making life better for you or for the people around you. Do you ever prepare a meal? Tidy up your bedroom? Go to work? Do some laundry? Hand in an assignment or work report? Each of these activities represents an accomplishment—a success that you can recognize and feel good about. Do you practice a musical instrument? Are you taking a course, doing a puzzle, or reading a book? These are all mastery activities that require sustained attention and effort.

Of course, if you're depressed, engaging in all these types of activities is even more difficult—and so it's an even greater accomplishment! For example, when Maya became depressed it was hard for her to find the energy to do regular housework and cooking. She decided that rather than being angry at herself for no longer keeping up her previous standards, she would feel good that despite her depression she was doing the dishes most nights and always had a hot meal for her children, even if it was a simple one.

Over the next week or so, see if you can notice and then record as many of your mastery and accomplishment activities as possible using the *My Current Mastery and Accomplishment Activities* worksheet that follows. Can you find at least one for each day? Then why not take a moment to pat yourself on the back and recognize your achievements? Perhaps you can even write "Well done!" in the margin beside each activity you recorded. Remember, when you're depressed, activities that were routine and easy before your depression may now represent real accomplishments.

My Current Mastery and Accomplishment Activities	
Date and time	Mastery and accomplishment activity

Now look over your worksheet and circle one or two activities that you could do a little more frequently. Focus especially on those activities that give you a strong feeling of mastery and accomplishment and that feel doable. You can also focus on any activities that are meaningful and consistent with your core values (see chapter 5). For example, Maya decided to focus on making her children's lunches before she went to bed.

What current mastery and accomplishment activities would you like to do more frequently? List them below.

_____

_____

_____

_____

_____

Do What's Worked in the Past

Earlier we asked you to reflect on some of the activities you used to do in the past that brought you a sense of mastery and accomplishment. Often, when depressed, we stop doing these activities or do them less often or with less care. These may be everyday activities such as getting to work on time or paying bills, or they may be activities with longer-term goals, like working toward a school diploma. Maya used to take great pride in how quickly she returned her students' homework. She believed it was important to give students immediate feedback. When she became depressed it was often weeks before she returned her students' homework and she no longer made any comments. She decided to make a plan to return homework more promptly and to write "Well done!" on the best assignments.

Think of some mastery and accomplishment activities that you have done in the past and would like to start doing again. Then write them down here.

_____

_____

_____

_____

_____

_____

It's important to note that when you are depressed you may not get as much of a sense of mastery and accomplishment from doing activities as you would have in the past. This is fairly common. However, what is crucial is taking the first step. If you stick with it, your sense of accomplishment will grow, and you may very well get more of a sense of mastery and accomplishment than you expect.

Supercharge Your Mastery and Accomplishment Activities with Your Values

In the previous chapter we supercharged Maya's enjoyable mood-boosting activities by linking them to her core values. We want to do the same for mood-boosting activities related to mastery and accomplishment. Let's look at an example. Ray, a client of Nina's, worked in a bank as an account manager. Work had been a struggle since they became depressed. Ray wanted to focus on completing an important work project as a mood-boosting activity related to feelings of mastery and accomplishment. Nina and Ray examined how Ray's values could supercharge completing the project.

Ray connected work to the value of financial and professional success. As a nonbinary Black person, they also valued being a mentor to younger racialized and LGBTQ+ colleagues. With this core value in mind, they decided to include mentoring younger team members as part of the project. After supercharging their mood-boosting activity with core values, Ray felt more motivated—and working on the project gave Ray even more of a sense of accomplishment.

Can you link the activities you identified as related to mastery and accomplishment to your core values? For example, if you identified cooking, is this related to the value of taking care of your health? Or maybe the value of friendship or family and creating welcoming and delicious meals? It could be that all of these values are important to you.

Look over the activities you just identified, both the activities you're already doing and would like to do more frequently and those you used to do but have stopped or are doing less often. Using the worksheet below, write down three or four of these activities that you would like to do more frequently or start doing. Now, take a moment to think about why they are important to you. What core values are they related to? We've added one of Ray's responses as an example.

Supercharge My Mastery and Accomplishment Activities with My Core Values	
Mastery and accomplishment activity	**Related core value**
Completing an important work project	Being a mentor and an example to junior racialized and LGBTQ+ colleagues

Let's reflect on the exercise you just did. What was it like to identify the values behind your mastery and accomplishment activities? How did it affect your motivation? How did it impact how you felt about completing the activities? Write down your thoughts here.

_____

_____

_____

_____

_____

Find New Mastery and Accomplishment Activities

Perhaps, like Ed, you're no longer physically capable of engaging in many of the activities that once gave you a sense of mastery and accomplishment. Or perhaps your life circumstances have changed in some way—you've retired, lost your job, moved—and you find yourself in a rut, lacking anything to do that gives you a sense of achievement. Whatever the reason, it could be time for you to consider taking on some new challenges, establishing new goals, and giving yourself some fresh opportunities to experience feelings of mastery and accomplishment. It may be hard to imagine, but it is possible that your depression could be an opportunity for new experiences and new growth.

When choosing new mastery and accomplishment activities to pursue it's important to keep your personal values squarely in mind. As an example, Stephen worked with a recent retiree who became depressed, in part because he no longer had work that challenged him or provided him with a sense of accomplishment. This individual strongly valued helping others. He decided to try volunteering for a local food bank. Not only did he enjoy himself and learn new skills but he also made a real contribution to his community.

For many people, volunteering or being active in organizations whose aim is to benefit others creates a great sense of both accomplishment and meaning. These organizations can be as varied as charitable organizations aimed at helping the homeless, political or religious organizations, or environmental organizations. What is important is that they be consistent with your values.

Look back on the personal values you identified in the previous chapter to remind yourself of what's really important to you. Now, choose two or three core values and ask yourself, *What activities could I do that are consistent with this value and would give me a sense of mastery and accomplishment?* Try to come up with some new mastery and accomplishment activities—big or small—that could be meaningful to you. Can you write them down below?

Core value: _____

What new mastery and accomplishment activity would be consistent with this value?

_____

_____

Core value: _____

What new mastery and accomplishment activity would be consistent with this value?

_____

_____

Core value: _____

What new mastery and accomplishment activity would be consistent with this value?

_____

_____

Since Ed was no longer able to derive a sense of mastery from his work as a carpenter, he began to look at other things he could do that would contribute to a sense of accomplishment and mastery. He decided to start with what had worked in the past, so he pushed himself to resume his furniture-making work. Even though he didn't get quite as much of a sense of accomplishment as he used to, he did get some. And, to Ed's surprise, he noticed that over time, as he stuck with it, he began to get more and more satisfaction from this work—especially when he saw the delight on Alex's face when he gave him a child-sized rocking chair built specially for him.

While Ed had to really push himself at first, he resumed washing his car on a weekly basis. He increasingly felt a sense of satisfaction and pride in his clean car, and it became easier to motivate himself to keep his car clean. Ed even started enjoying going out for drives once again.

Being a hard worker was one of Ed's important personal values. When he was unable to work as a carpenter, his self-esteem plummeted. Stephen and Ed began to look for new ways for Ed to work hard and to be productive—without the risk of reinjuring himself. After considering a number of options, Ed decided to improve his skills in reading blueprints and estimating materials and prices for large construction projects so he could work as an estimator. Ed started a retraining course. While he often found it hard to keep motivated, he felt good to be learning again and to be productive.

What About You?

Now we'd like you to focus on one or two of the mastery and accomplishment activities that you've identified throughout this chapter. It could be something you're doing now that you'd like to do more of. Or it could be something that you've done in the past that you'd like to resume. Perhaps it's one of the brand-new mastery or accomplishment activities that you came up with after reflecting on what else you could do.

If you're having a hard time coming up with ideas, ask yourself what advice you would give a friend. You may also find it useful to talk to other people you know—ideally those who share at least some of your values, or who know you well. What are they doing that gives them a sense of mastery and accomplishment? Do they have any ideas for you? Don't worry about getting it perfect. Come at this with the mindset of "Let's try it and see what happens!"

Now let's see if you can make a plan. You can use the *Action Plan* worksheet below. Make sure your plan is specific and doable, and can be part of your routine. As always, it's also helpful to consider first steps, and to anticipate any obstacles you may encounter in moving forward with your mastery and accomplishment activities.

Action Plan: Mastery and Accomplishment Activities				
What I'll do	Is my plan...	My first step	Obstacles I may encounter	How I'll handle these obstacles
	☐ specific? ☐ doable? ☐ part of my routine?			
	☐ specific? ☐ doable? ☐ part of my routine?			
	☐ specific? ☐ doable? ☐ part of my routine?			
	☐ specific? ☐ doable? ☐ part of my routine?			

Take a moment to sit back, take a few deep breaths, and rehearse your plans in your imagination. Remember to make them as detailed as possible. Now, rehearse your plans another two times. Often the more we rehearse in our imagination, the more doable our plans start to feel.

Now it's time to implement your plans. Don't forget to rate your moods before and after engaging in your mastery and accomplishment activity. You can use the *Rate My Mood* worksheet from chapter 3. Notice any increase in your positive moods and give yourself a smile. If your mood didn't improve, keep at it. It can take a while to see your mood improve. How could you make the activity even more of a mood booster?

_____

_____

_____

_____

One last thought. It's nice to experience success, but how you get there is also really important. Try to take some satisfaction and pride in the steps you are taking, no matter how small. After all, each of those steps is a big success in itself! If you focus on the journey, getting to the destination will often take care of itself.

What's Next?

Take a moment to think about what you want to take from this chapter. What did you learn that might help you have a better life and get over your depression?

_____

_____

_____

_____

How could you make a plan to bring what was meaningful to you in the chapter into your own life?

_____

_____

_____

Take a look at the illustration below for an overview of what we've covered in this chapter. Does anything stick out that you want to focus on in the next few days? How could you make a plan to incorporate it into your life?

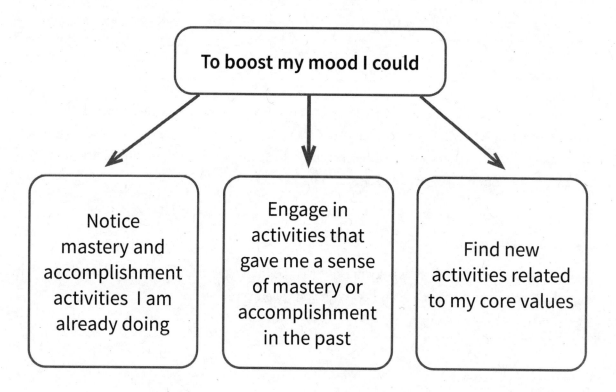

Figure 6.2: Effective Mood-Boosting Behavior: Mastery and Accomplishment

In the next chapter, we're going to give you some powerful tools for overcoming depression-related avoidance—including procrastination—and equip you with strategies for facing and solving your problems more effectively. Let's do it!

CHAPTER 7

Stop Avoiding—Learn to Face and Solve Your Problems

When we're depressed, we tend to want to avoid situations that we think will be stressful or challenging. While avoiding problems can bring a short-lived sense of relief, avoidance rarely leads to productive solutions, and inevitably makes our problems—and our moods—much, much worse.

Avoiding our problems leads to an avoidance trap, a vicious cycle in which the more we avoid, the worse we feel—and the worse we feel, the more we avoid. It starts to feel impossible to face and solve our problems or even just find a better way to cope. It can start to feel pretty hopeless. The illustration below demonstrates how avoidance traps work.

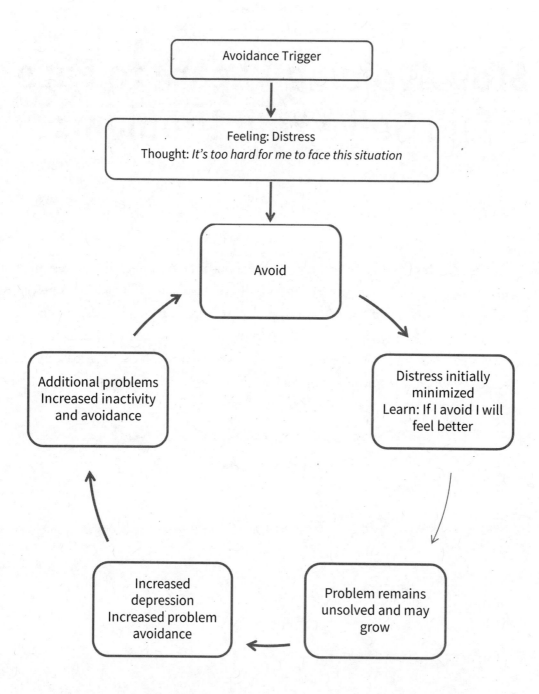

Figure 7.1: How the Avoidance Trap Works

Identify Your Avoidance Triggers

Let's start with learning how to identify avoidance triggers. Avoidance triggers are situations or tasks we find difficult, uncomfortable, or stressful in some way, and that we therefore want to avoid—even though our lives would be much better if we didn't. We all have avoidance triggers: the household chores we dislike; the pile of paper on our desk that just seems to keep growing; the difficult conversation we need to have with someone; or the task that we think will be hard or upsetting. Of course, when we're depressed, everything seems more difficult, and we may be tempted to avoid even tasks that normally would be easy. Often self-care activities like making a dentist's appointment, getting a haircut, or taking a shower can start to feel difficult. The list of potential avoidance triggers is endless.

When I (Nina) asked Maya what she was avoiding, Maya sighed, looked down, and said, "I'm not sure that I've taken care of all the taxes related to my mother's estate. I'm actually not all that clear on what needs to be done." I asked if there was anything else she was avoiding. Maya sighed again and said, "I guess I'm avoiding seeing my friends." When I (Stephen) asked Ed if he was avoiding anything, Ed raised his eyebrows and said, "Well, sure, I guess we all know I am really out of shape. I've been avoiding any kind of exercise." He paused, and then continued hesitantly, "You could also say I'm avoiding thinking about what's next. This hand pain thing could be around for a while."

Ask yourself, *What situations or tasks do I tend to avoid?* List them here:

_____

_____

_____

_____

This coming week, notice which situations or tasks trigger a desire to avoid, and then add them to your list.

Recognize Your Avoidance Patterns

There are many, many ways to avoid. We're going to list some of the most common ways of avoiding and then ask you to identify your own avoidance patterns.

Procrastinating

Procrastination is one of the more obvious forms of avoidance. Here's a list of some of the things that our clients—and if we're being completely honest, we ourselves—tend to put off. As you read through the list, try to think of examples from your own life.

- Unpaid bills

- Reading and sending emails

- Making important phone calls

- School or work projects

- Paperwork, especially if left on desks and tables

- Tasks related to children, the house, the car, or other personal matters

- Tasks related to organizing, cleaning, repairing, or neatening up

- Tasks related to personal care—doctor's appointments, haircuts, exercise

- Making dates to see friends and family

What do you put off? What are the activities or tasks that you know are important but that you never seem to get around to doing? Write them below:

_____

_____

_____

_____

Sleeping or "Resting"

If you are tired and you sleep, you generally wake up feeling refreshed. However, sleeping, and even feelings of tiredness, can actually be a way of avoiding difficult or distressing situations. Ask yourself, *Do I give in to feeling tired and go to bed when I'd promised myself I would do an unpleasant task?* If the answer is yes, you may be using sleep or resting as a way of avoiding.

Think of a time when you started to feel tired and decided to rest. What activities were you doing, or had you planned on doing?

_____

_____

Engaging in Distracting Activities

Do you avoid important but unpleasant tasks by doing other things that are easier for you? For example, when Maya thought about doing financial tasks related to her mother's estate, she would get busy with doing something for her children. These were important tasks, but she never got around to handling the financial issues related to her mother's estate. My (Nina) favorite form of distraction is checking text messages when I'm in the middle of writing—especially if the writing is not going so well! I (Stephen) suddenly become very interested in straightening pictures on the wall when I'm facing the task of sorting through and filing the piles of documents and papers that accumulate on my desk.

What do you do to distract yourself from tasks you may find difficult or hard to face?

_____

_____

_____

_____

Ruminating, Worrying, and Complaining

Productive thinking about problems or tasks you need to take care of is important and helpful. However, *ruminating* (that is, having constant, repetitive thoughts about a situation) and worrying are rarely productive and can be a way of avoiding having to make a decision or take action.

Complaining can also be helpful at times. Sharing your problems and challenges with friends and family can be useful. However, if you always complain but never change what you do, then complaining can become a way of avoiding taking action on problems or difficult situations in your life.

What are the situations you complain, worry, or ruminate about, but don't act on?

_____

_____

_____

"Forgetting"

Forgetting about a task or a problem can be a way of avoiding. Do you "forget" about some problems—remembering them only when you are not able to do anything about them? A client of Nina's needed to have a difficult phone conversation with a family member. Coincidentally, they only "remembered" to call the person when they were in the middle of putting the kids to bed, in a work meeting, or at night when it was too late to call.

What are some situations that you "forget" about until you are not able to act on them?

_____

_____

_____

Self-Numbing: Alcohol, Drugs, Bingeing (Food, TV, Internet)

Many of us occasionally engage in mindless activities when we want to relax. That's pretty normal and can even be helpful at times. However, if these mindless activities become excessive or are used as a way of avoiding tasks or problems, they can be counterproductive.

What are the difficult situations you avoid by numbing yourself?

_____

_____

_____

_____

How do you tend to numb yourself?

_____

_____

Before we move on, take a moment to look over the ways of avoiding you just read about. If you can think of any we missed, list them here:

_____

_____

_____

_____

Face Your Challenges

It's now time to get yourself out of your avoidance traps by making specific plans to face the situations you've been avoiding. We think you will find that this is a powerful mood-boosting strategy. Even though it may seem daunting at first, once you start it will be easier than you think.

When Ed first decided he wanted to start washing his car again, he found that other things always seemed to come up and he kept "forgetting" to do it. So, Ed decided to make a specific plan. He made a commitment to washing the car on Saturday at 2:00 p.m. He wrote "Wash the car" into his electronic calendar, and even programmed his phone to send him a reminder at 1:45. Maya realized she had been numbing herself with binge watching a Netflix series at night rather than grading papers. She made a plan to grade five papers a night, three nights a week.

In the worksheet that follows, start by listing two or three situations you are avoiding. They can be the same as the avoidance triggers you identified earlier on. Then, as you've done previously, make a plan to face those situations—a plan that is specific and doable, and can be part of your routine. Be sure to identify the first step.

Action Plan: Face My Challenges

What I'll do	Is my plan...	My first step	Obstacles I may encounter	How I'll handle these obstacles
	☐ specific? ☐ doable? ☐ part of my routine?			
	☐ specific? ☐ doable? ☐ part of my routine?			
	☐ specific? ☐ doable? ☐ part of my routine?			
	☐ specific? ☐ doable? ☐ part of my routine?			

Take a moment to imagine accomplishing the plan you made. In your mind's eye, see yourself carrying out your plan in as much detail as possible. Now give yourself an imaginary pat on the back. Tell yourself, *It's hard to face what you are avoiding, so good work in making a plan.* Take a breath and now tell yourself, *You can do it!* Now, ask yourself if you would like to change anything in your plan. Imagine making the changes you would like. Then practice two more times.

Now you're ready to take action on your plan. Start by committing yourself to taking the first step. Once you've completed the first step, rate your mood using the *Rate My Mood* worksheet from chapter 3—then take a moment to congratulate yourself. Finally, pause and notice how nice it feels to face rather than avoid the challenges in your life.

Find Solutions to Your Problems

Life can be very complex and challenging at times. Sometimes we are tempted to avoid situations because we're just not sure how to handle them. For Maya, dealing with the financial issues from her mother's estate and reaching out to old friends would be examples. We may also face difficult situations we have no direct control over (for example, a chronic medical condition, the loss of a close relationship, systemic discrimination). In these types of situations the question becomes how to respond to and manage the situation.

When we face difficult situations we can get caught in a problem-solving rut, trying the same ineffective solutions over and over. In this section we want to teach you a problem-solving approach that is backed by solid research (Cuijpers et al. 2020). It will help you step back, see your problems in a different light, and open up solutions you may not have thought of.

There are six steps to problem solving. You can use this very silly ditty to remember them— "IBC and PPE can help ME" (we know—totally ridiculous—but we like it!)

I=Identify a problem	**P** =Plan your solution
B=Brainstorm different solutions	**P**=Proceed with your solution
C=Choose a solution to try	**E**=Evaluate

Identify a Problem

Even if you have a lot of problems, it's important to focus on just *one* at a time. It's difficult to deal with multiple problems all at once.

Maya chose to focus on the problem of reconnecting with Sharon, an old friend she had lost contact with since she became depressed. Sharon had sent her a few messages about six months ago, but Maya had never responded. Now she felt awkward about reaching out and contacting Sharon.

Now it's your turn. Think of a problem that you've been avoiding and want to work on. Since this may be your first time problem solving, choose a problem that is of easy-to-moderate difficulty. Once you understand problem solving, you can try the approach with more difficult problems.

Write your problem here: _____

_____

Brainstorm Different Solutions

The next step in a problem-solving approach involves brainstorming a list of potential solutions. When brainstorming, the goal is to think of as many different types of solutions as you possibly can *without judging your ideas*. It doesn't matter if your ideas are good, bad, silly, or great. Later you will evaluate your ideas, but not now. Include a few far-fetched and seemingly impossible solutions—they can inspire you to think outside the box. At times combining a really far-fetched idea with something more conventional can result in a surprisingly creative and effective solution.

Sometimes it may be hard to come up with solutions—even far-fetched ones. Below are some questions you can ask yourself to help generate new ideas. You may want to use the *Brainstorming Questions* worksheet below. Focus on the problem you identified earlier and try to answer all the questions. There may be some overlap in your answers; don't worry about that—it's fine. We've included some of Maya's answers to these questions as an illustration.

Brainstorming Questions

Problem: Maya: Reconnecting with Sharon—whom I've ignored for six months

Me:

What are some different ways I could handle this problem?	Maya: Just text Sharon and ask how she is. I could also check her Facebook page and get a sense of how she was doing.
	Me:
How have I handled similar situations in the past?	Maya: I have texted my friend, asked how they are, said I had been really busy, that I felt bad I had not returned their messages, and suggested we get together.
	Me:
What would I suggest to someone else (maybe a close friend or a relative) who had this problem?	Maya: I might suggest that they text their friend and honestly tell them that they had been depressed and that was why they had been out of touch.
	Me:
What do I think someone who cared for me would suggest if they knew I had this problem?	Maya: They might suggest that I check Sharon's Facebook page and leave a message.
	Me:

Is there any information I'm ignoring that could be helpful?	Maya: Sharon has been a good friend for a long time and would understand that I had been depressed. She would probably want to see me.
	Me:
If there is an aspect of the problem that I cannot change and must accept. Can I think of coping strategies?	Maya: I have to accept that I did not get back to her for six months, and she might be upset. To cope, I can remind myself that it's not the end of the world if she's upset and she'll probably get over it. I want to try and not take this personally. It's not because I was a bad person, but because I was depressed that I did not get back to her.
	Me:
If I acted according to my core values, what solutions would come to mind?	Maya: I really value our friendship and I would want to reach out to her.
	Me:
Is there someone I could turn to for advice who might be helpful?	Maya: I am not sure. Maybe my cousin who generally has good ideas and has met Sharon.
	Me:

Based on your answers to the questions above, write down some possible solutions. Remember to include even far-fetched or silly solutions.

_____

_____

_____

_____

_____

Choose a Solution to Try

When Maya looked at her list of possible solutions she wasn't sure which one to choose. I (Nina) showed her the _Weigh the Pros and Cons_ worksheet. It involves choosing two or three solutions from your brainstorming list that seem the best to you, and then identifying the advantages and disadvantages of each solution.

Maya chose three possible solutions: (1) check Sharon's Facebook page to see what was happening in Sharon's life; (2) text Sharon that she had been depressed and suggest that they get together; and (3) text Sharon that she had been busy, that she felt bad about not being in contact, and suggest they get together. Here is Maya's _Weigh the Pros and Cons_ worksheet.

Weigh the Pros and Cons		
Possible solutions	**Pros/advantages**	**Cons/disadvantages**
1. Check Sharon's Facebook page	Very low risk It would be at least something I could start with I could find out if there was anything new in her life	It won't help me connect with Sharon.
2. Text Sharon that I have been depressed and suggest that we get together.	Sharon would understand why I had been out of touch. Sharon would feel empathy for me.	I would feel very vulnerable telling her about my depression. If Sharon did not respond I would be very embarrassed. I would be very anxious.
3. Text Sharon that I have been busy, that I feel bad that I have not been in contact, and suggest we get together.	Feels low risk Easy to do Good chance Sharon would respond	Sharon might not understand why we haven't been in touch and not get back to me. Sharon might be angry with me for not getting back to her earlier. I would be a bit anxious.

When Maya looked at the pros and cons, she decided that, although texting Sharon to tell her that she had been busy wasn't a perfect solution, it was the best one she had come up with thus far and she was willing to try it. She decided that she would also check Sharon's Facebook page as a good way to ease herself into making contact with Sharon again.

Now take a look at the potential solutions you listed earlier and choose two or three that appeal to you. Like Maya, you may want to combine a few. Then complete the blank *Weigh the Pros and Cons* worksheet that follows.

Weigh the Pros and Cons		
Possible solutions	**Pros/advantages**	**Cons/disadvantages**

Look over the advantages and disadvantages of each of your potential solutions. Don't expect an ideal solution. Choose the best one, or the one you would like to try—and let's make a plan.

Plan Your Solution

After you've chosen a potential solution, the next step is to develop your action plan. Remember, you want your plan to be specific and doable. It's also important to identify the first step, and to anticipate and address any obstacles you may encounter. Let's look at Maya's solution. Maya thought she could easily check Sharon's Facebook page and made a plan to be sure it happened. She then made a plan to text Sharon.

Action Plan: Problem Solving				
What I'll do	**Is my plan...**	**My first step**	**Obstacles I may encounter**	**How I'll handle these obstacles**
Check Sharon's Facebook page at 2:30 this afternoon	☑ specific? ☑ doable? ☑ part of my routine?	Clear time to go on Facebook	None	N/A
Text Sharon at 3:00 p.m. and suggest we get together	☑ specific? ☑ doable? ☑ part of my routine?	Write message	I will feel anxious Plan	Remind myself I want to do this, that I care about my friendship with Sharon

Now it's your turn to plan your solution. This can be a difficult step to complete. You may have to push yourself a bit, but once it's done, your plan will feel much more doable. Complete the *Action Plan: Problem Solving* worksheet for the solution you chose.

Action Plan: Problem Solving				
What I'll do	**Is my plan...**	**My first step**	**Obstacles I may encounter**	**How I'll handle these obstacles**
	☐ specific? ☐ doable? ☐ part of my routine?			
	☐ specific? ☐ doable? ☐ part of my routine?			
	☐ specific? ☐ doable? ☐ part of my routine?			
	☐ specific? ☐ doable? ☐ part of my routine?			

Now take a moment to go over your plan in your imagination. Sit back and visualize yourself implementing your plan step by step, in as much detail as possible. Ask yourself if there is anything you can do to increase your chances of success. Make any changes to your plan that will help you succeed, then go through it two more times in your imagination.

Proceed and Evaluate the Outcome

Now it's time to put your plan into action. Don't forget, depression will do everything it can to encourage you to avoid your problems. This means you may find it hard to put your plan into action. That's normal. Just keep trying!

It's important to evaluate the effectiveness of your solution after you've tried it. Sometimes our plans are only moderately successful, and occasionally they don't work out at all. Human problems can be tough to solve and may require a few tries. Don't be discouraged. It's important to evaluate the outcome and keep trying.

In Maya's case, her plan went well. It was easy for Maya to check Sharon's Facebook page. She still felt really anxious about texting Sharon, but she pushed herself. Sharon got back to her almost immediately and was happy to get together. Maya and Sharon planned a lunch for the following week.

Think of your plan as an experiment. You want to try your plan and then evaluate the outcome. How did it go? Were you able to face and solve your problem? If so, congratulations! You can use the same approach to deal with other problems in your life. If your plan did not go well, don't be discouraged. Just ask yourself a few questions:

In what way did the plan go well?

_____

_____

_____

What part of the plan did not go well?

_____

_____

_____

How can I improve the plan and try it again?

_____

_____

_____

_____

Now that I have tried one solution, is there a different solution I want to try?

_____

_____

_____

_____

Even if your initial solution didn't work out as you had hoped, the important thing is to keep at it. We know you can do it.

What's Next?

It's time to take a moment and reflect on what has been meaningful to you in this chapter. What did you learn that might help you have a better life and get over your depression?

_____

_____

_____

How can you bring what was meaningful to you in the chapter into your own life? What are your thoughts about making a plan?

_____

_____

_____

In this section of the book, we've focused on identifying and incorporating a range of important mood-boosting activities into your regular routine. We've also discussed how to face and solve your problems. This illustration presents an overview of what we've covered.

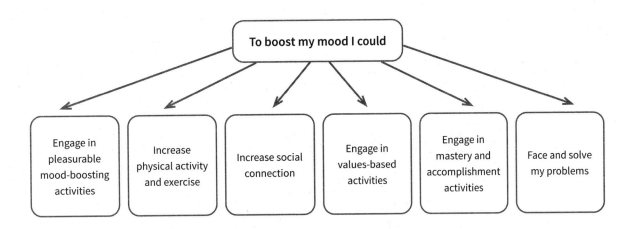

Figure 7.2: Overview of Effective Mood-Boosting Activities

We've come a long way. However, there's a catch: when we're depressed it can be very hard to find the motivation to get going and to stay going. It's just what depression does to us. However, much like a muscle, motivation can be exercised and strengthened. In the next section of this workbook, we're going to introduce you to a number of powerful strategies to help you build your motivation muscle so that it's easier to add mood-boosting activities to your life. We'll start with showing you how to use behavioral principles to overcome the lethargy of depression, strengthen your motivation, and get rolling. Let's get to it!

PART THREE

Jumpstart Your Motivation

CHAPTER 8

Behavioral Strategies for Getting Going

Depression robs us of our get-up-and-go and makes us feel lethargic, tired, and apathetic.

When we introduce behavioral activation to our depressed clients they often say something like, "I know that engaging in mood-boosting activities would be really helpful for me, but I just need to feel more motivated before I can get started."

The idea that we have to feel motivated before taking action seems logical enough—but it's a fallacy. If you wait until you *feel* motivated before taking your first step, you'll probably be waiting for a long, long time! The truth of the matter is that we begin to feel motivated and have more energy *after* we've started doing an activity—not the other way around. As the illustration below shows, this is another self-reinforcing cycle—increased activity leads to increased motivation, and increased motivation leads to increased activity.

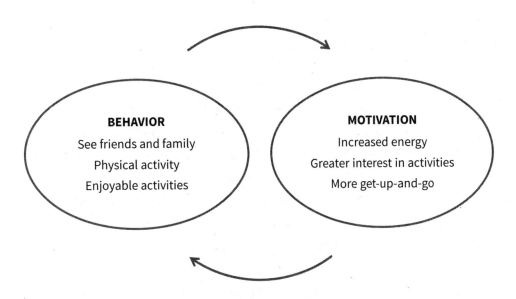

Figure 8.1: The Positive Cycle of Behavior and Motivation

Think of mood-boosting activities as your medicine. When you're sick you don't ask yourself, *Do I feel like taking my medicine today?* You just take it. When it comes to engaging in mood-boosting activities, a lot of our clients find it helpful to tell themselves, *Just do it!* Don't let your depressed feelings boss you around. Don't wait to feel motivated. *Just do it!*

What About You?

Choose a mood-boosting activity that you've been having a hard time starting. Take a moment and make a commitment to yourself to carry through on your mood-boosting plan. Try standing tall, looking straight ahead, and announcing your plan to yourself out loud. Write it down on a sticky note and place it on the fridge or make it your phone's wallpaper, or just write it down here:

My plan is to _____

_____

This is your *Don't Wait—Just Do It* plan.

Target Your Low-Motivation Times

Everyone's level of motivation varies over the course of the day. For many people suffering from depression, mornings are a particularly tough time to get going. Ed would wake up in the morning and lie in bed feeling more and more depressed, finding it harder and harder to get on with his day. Other people find that the afternoon or evening is a time when they are stuck in this pattern of depressive "do-nothingism." The best thing you can do is identify and plan for these times.

Ed made a plan for the morning—his low-motivation time. His plan started with setting an alarm and getting up, rather than lying in bed and ruminating. He decided that when the alarm went off he would throw off the covers and sit up. After that, he planned on washing his face and brushing his teeth. Then he could have his morning cup of coffee.

Again, do anything that just gets you moving. It doesn't have to be perfect—start with where you are. For example, Ed was sleeping until 9:00 a.m., then lying in bed until 10 a.m. He decided to set an alarm for 9:15, even though ideally he wanted to get up a bit earlier.

Often when you add simple get-going activities to your low-motivation part of the day you have more energy and motivation for the rest of the day as well.

What About You?

Try to identify your own low-motivation part of the day. Below, we've provided you with a *Target Your Low-Motivation Times* worksheet. You can use it to plan get-going activities to boost your motivation during the times when you feel stuck. They don't have to be big or complicated. Almost anything that gets you moving will do—we'd encourage you to keep it simple and easy. The key is to have a very specific plan for your difficult times of the day.

Try this experiment. Using this worksheet, make a note of your level of motivation before you engage in your get-going activities, and then note your level of motivation afterward. You can see Ed's example below.

Notice what happens. Did your motivation increase even a little?

Target My Low Motivation Times			
Low-motivation times	Get-going activities	Motivation before 1 (very little) to 10 (a lot)	Motivation after 1 (very little) to 10 (a lot)
Morning, lying in bed	Get out of bed Wash my face Brush my teeth Make a cup of coffee	3	6

Remember, you'll get a motivation boost from doing any kind of activity—anything to get yourself moving. These motivation-boosting activities may not be hugely important or meaningful in and of themselves, but if they create even a tiny bit of movement for you, that may be good enough to get you rolling.

Break Things Down into Small, Manageable Steps

When we're depressed, getting started on mood-boosting activities can feel overwhelming. Even small tasks or problems can feel big and complicated. One way to get going on tasks that feel overwhelming is to break them down into much smaller, more manageable steps. You can then tackle each step one by one in a logical order. Psychologists call this technique "graded task assignment."

Here's an example. One of my (Stephen's) clients, Chris, was in their mid-fifties and had been depressed for the past year. They had been avoiding cleaning their house for several months and wanted to clean their fridge. However, the thought of all the work involved was completely overwhelming. Chris and I began by breaking the task of cleaning the fridge into a series of small, manageable steps. Chris thought of starting by locating some paper towels and spray cleaner, and then cleaning out the butter shelf in the fridge. Chris then identified a number of other small steps and placed them in a logical order. I encouraged Chris to create a schedule for each of these tasks and to estimate how much time each would take. You can see Chris's plan in this *Break It Down* worksheet.

Break It Down	
Activity: *Clean out the fridge*	
Smaller steps	**When?** **For how long?**
1. Locate paper towels and spray cleaner.	Monday afternoon at 2:00 p.m. 5 minutes
2. Remove butter from butter shelf. Clean the butter shelf, then replace butter.	Monday afternoon at 2:15 p.m. 10 minutes
3. Find a food-waste bin.	Tuesday morning at 10:00 a.m. 5 minutes
4. Remove food items from the vegetable crisper, place old or rotten food items in waste bin, clean crisper, and put fresh items back into crisper.	Tuesday morning at 10:15 a.m. 15 minutes
5. Remove food items from the upper shelf, place old or rotten items in waste bin, clean upper shelf, and replace fresh items.	Wednesday afternoon at 2:00 p.m. 15 minutes
6. Remove food items from the lower shelf, place old or rotten items in waste bin, clean lower shelf, and replace fresh items.	Thursday morning at 9:00 a.m. 15 minutes

When you're depressed, even small everyday tasks can seem huge and daunting. For Chris, the idea of cleaning out the fridge seemed completely overwhelming at first. However, by breaking it down into steps, it seemed more manageable, and Chris felt motivated to get started.

The next week Chris reported that the butter dish was clean and even a bit more of the fridge had been cleaned. Chris and I checked that the rest of the tasks were doable. Starting to clean the fridge gave Chris a real mood boost and increased their motivation to take on other tasks.

A heads-up: It can be hard to plan out a whole task. Sometimes it's easier to plan the first few steps, and once they are done, then plan the next steps.

What About You?

Try to think of an activity, a task, or a goal that feels big and overwhelming and that you are having trouble getting started on. Now, use this blank worksheet to break it down into small, manageable steps. Don't forget to schedule each step and estimate how long you think it will take. Notice whether you feel more motivated once you have broken the task down into specific steps. Remember, you can just plan the first few steps; you don't have to plan the whole task.

Break It Down	
Activity:	
Smaller steps	**When?** **For how long?**

Now start with the first step. Once that's done, give yourself a pat on the back and ask yourself, *What's the next step?* Then do that step. Before you know it, you'll have done much more than you would have ever thought possible!

Use Positive Reinforcement

Psychologists know that if something positive happens to you after you engage in an activity, you will be more likely to do that activity again. This is called "positive reinforcement." For example, if we complete a task and then receive a hug, or someone says we did a good job, or we receive a bonus, or we feel appreciated, we are being positively reinforced for that activity. It's very likely that we'll feel more motivated to do the same task again. We may even be motivated to engage in similar types of activities.

We can't usually control how much other people positively reinforce us, but we can reward ourselves for the things we do—thereby creating our own positive reinforcement and increasing our motivation to do the activity again. We are going to show you how to positively reinforce yourself for engaging in mood-boosting activities—especially those activities that you find hard to motivate yourself to do.

Maya thought it would help her depression if she saw more friends and went out more.

However, she wasn't sure why, but she was having a really hard time even texting her friends to suggest getting together. I (Nina) explained positive reinforcement. Maya was curious and wanted to see if positive reinforcement would increase her motivation.

Maya decided that she would text her friend Joanne to see how she was doing and suggest a coffee date. I asked Maya if she could think of something really nice she could do for herself after sending the text, as a reward for having had the courage to contact Joanne. At first Maya had trouble coming up with ideas, but eventually she decided on two rewards. First, she would write herself a note congratulating herself for challenging herself and doing something difficult. Second, she would treat herself to a specialty coffee that she loved, but that was a bit too expensive to buy regularly.

At our next session, Maya happily told me that she had contacted Joanne and arranged a coffee date for next week. Maya thought that looking forward to the positive reinforcements had given her a motivational boost to contact Joanne. After Joanne's positive response, plus the positive reinforcement she gave herself, Maya felt more motivated to contact other friends.

What About You?

Let's look at how you can use positive reinforcement to improve your motivation.

First, identify an activity that you want to incorporate into your behavioral activation plan.

_____

Next, see if you can come up with some tangible rewards that you can use to reinforce yourself after engaging in this activity. Take a look at the list below for some ideas. Make the reward as specific and concrete as possible. Be sure to choose a positive reinforcer that is something that you really like, that makes you feel good or is special in some way. It could be words of affirmation and praise, or it could be a treat of some sort.

Here are a few ideas of positive reinforcers; see if you can come up with some more!

- Do something fun that you often don't have time for.

- Take yourself out to your favorite restaurant.

- Make yourself a nice cup of tea, coffee, or hot chocolate.

- Enjoy a bubble bath.

- Treat yourself to a candy bar.

- Have a specialty coffee.

- Go to see a movie.

- Watch an episode of your favorite TV series.

- Go to bed early.

- Put some money into your vacation fund jar.

- Play a video game.

- Get a massage.

- Give yourself some free time.

- Look yourself in the mirror and say to yourself, "Good job!"

What else? Take a moment to jot down some other reinforcers you could use.

_____

_____

_____

When you reward yourself for engaging in mood-boosting activities, you also increase the overall amount of positive reinforcement in your life—which is likely to boost your motivation and generally help you feel better.

Use the Premack Principle

The Premack Principle (Herrod at al. 2022; Premack, 1959) is a technique that is similar to positive reinforcement, but with an interesting twist. It involves identifying activities that you know are important, but that you don't feel all that motivated to do. You then pair them with activities you engage in regularly and that you like or are at least somewhat pleasant for you—for example, watching a particular series, eating dinner, playing video games, or using social media.

When we use the Premack Principle, we allow ourselves to engage in regular, relatively pleasant or enjoyable activities only *after* we complete the behavioral activation tasks that we've been avoiding or finding hard to get started on. In a sense, we "borrow" the motivation we already have for the more pleasant activities that we engage in regularly to help us get started on things that don't come as easily.

Here's an example of how I (Stephen) used the Premack Principle. I don't really enjoy mowing the lawn all that much—it's a bit of a chore for me—and I was having a hard time getting down to it. As a diehard football fan, I regularly watch NFL games at 1:00 p.m. every Sunday. I made a deal with myself. Before sitting down to watch the game on Sunday, I would first mow the lawn. Guess what? I mowed the lawn! Then I enjoyed watching the game—and felt good about mowing the lawn as well.

What About You?

Now it's your turn to try the Premack Principle. Let's take it step by step. First, identify an activity that you'd like to incorporate into your life, but which you find hard to get motivated to do. We'll call this your "hard-to-start" activity. It could be one of the mood-boosting behaviors we've discussed earlier in this book.

My hard-to-start activity is: _____

Second, identify an activity that you engage in frequently and find at least somewhat pleasant. We'll call this your "regular-and-pleasant" activity.

My regular-and-pleasant activity is: _____

Third, make a deal with yourself to engage in your regular-and-pleasant activity only after you do your hard-to-start activity. We call this a "first-then" deal. For me, the deal was "*First* mow the lawn, *then* watch NFL football." Here's example from Nina's life: "*First* do fifteen minutes of exercise in the morning, *then* have your coffee." The more enjoyable your regular-and-pleasant activity is, the more effective your first-then deal will be.

Write down your "first-then" deal here: _____

Fourth—and finally—make a plan for your hard-to-start activity.

Were you able to use the Premack Principle to get started on one of your mood-boosting activities? If so, congratulations (that was a positive reinforcer by the way)! You'll find that it's easier and easier to get yourself started on important activities the more you practice the Premack Principle. If you weren't able to do it, don't worry. It's not always as easy as it sounds—especially when you're depressed. The important thing is to keep trying. Also, start small—make sure your hard-to-start activity is doable, and that you have a clear first step and a good plan.

What's Next?

Look over this chapter. What was relevant to increasing your motivation? Which of the strategies we covered resonate with you most strongly?

_____

_____

_____

In the illustration below, you can find a summary of what we covered. What ideas from this chapter would you like to try in your own life? Would you like to make a plan?

_____

_____

_____

_____

_____

_____

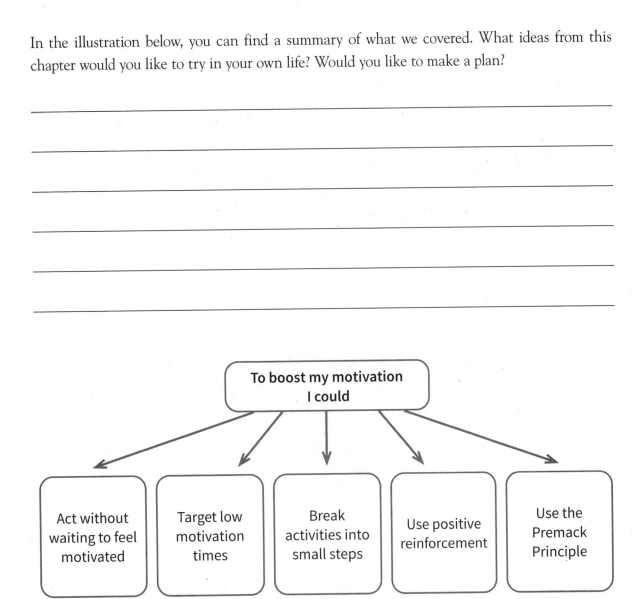

Figure 8.2: Behavioral Strategies for Boosting Motivation

In the next chapter we're going to look at how the way you think can play into feelings of depression and low motivation. Then, we're going to look at how you can develop thinking patterns that will increase your motivation and get you—and keep you—going with your behavioral activation plans. Let's give that some thought!

CHAPTER 9

Thoughts Can Boost Your Motivation and Improve Your Mood

Up to this point, we've focused primarily on how what we do—our behavior—affects our mood and our motivation. But the way we think plays a key role in depression as well. When we're depressed, we get stuck in negative thinking patterns that not only make us feel bad but also drain our motivation for taking positive, mood-boosting action.

Let's look at some of Maya's motivation-busting thoughts. Maya had planned to walk with her colleague Alicia during her lunch hour. When it was time to go, Maya started telling herself things like *I'll have nothing to say*; *I'm too tired*; and *I won't enjoy the walk anyhow*. Feeling depressed, she texted Alicia and canceled their walk. Maya's negative, motivation-zapping thoughts played a big role in her decision to avoid walking with Alicia. The illustration below shows how Maya's motivation-busting thoughts set up a vicious cycle that kept her trapped in her low mood and lack of motivation.

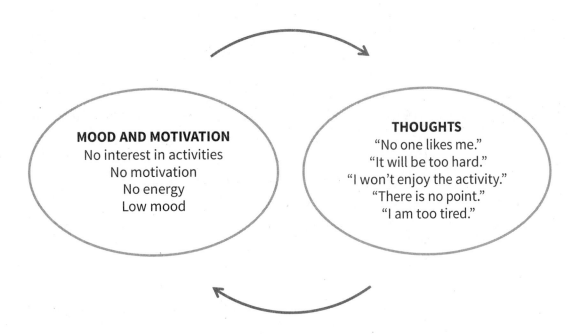

Figure 9.1: The Vicious Cycle of Negative Thinking and Low Motivation/Mood

In this chapter we'll show you how to identify and challenge your motivation-busting thoughts, and help you transform them into thoughts that will improve your mood and motivate you to get going with your behavioral activation plans.

Identify Your Motivation-Busting Thinking Traps

Depression lies to us. It tries to get us to believe, for example, that change is impossible, that the future is completely hopeless, and that we are inadequate. Not only are these kinds of thoughts untrue, but they're extremely unhelpful—they make us feel sad, despondent, and unmotivated (Josefowitz and Myran 2021).

Depression's motivation-busting lies fall into a number of very predictable patterns that psychologists call "cognitive distortions" or "thinking traps." Although there are many thinking traps associated with depression, we're going to focus on five of them that are particularly important in demotivating us from taking steps toward building a better life. They're called "fortune-telling," "catastrophizing," "mind reading," "should statements," and "emotional reasoning." As we go through each of these traps, see if you can recognize any of them in your own thinking patterns.

Fortune-Telling

When we engage in fortune-telling, we believe that we know with certainty what the future holds *and* that it's bleak. When you're caught in this thinking trap you may be convinced, for example, that you won't enjoy any of your mood-boosting activities, that nothing you do will help you feel better, or that no matter what you do, your future will be filled with failure and misery. Fortune-telling leads to feelings of hopelessness and apathy. It's easy to see how having these types of thoughts can seriously undermine motivation for mood-boosting activities.

Can you think of an example of fortune-telling from your own life? Write it down here:

_____

Catastrophizing

Fortune-telling often goes together with another thinking trap that we call "catastrophizing." When we catastrophize, we view our worst-case scenario as being highly likely and believe that if it should occur, it would be absolutely terrible—the end of the world. An example of catastrophizing would be assuming that if you make one mistake, people will lose all respect for you, you'll fail at school, or you'll lose your job. For many people, catastrophic thoughts are accompanied by vivid mental images of the catastrophic event occurring. Catastrophizing is a motivation zapper because it creates feelings of fear and helplessness about potential outcomes, leaving us feeling paralyzed and overwhelmed.

Can you think of an example of catastrophizing from your own life? Write it down here:

_____

Mind Reading

When we engage in mind reading, we assume that we know *for sure* what other people are feeling and thinking *and* that they are thinking negative things about us. For example, without evidence, we interpret other people's behavior as an indication that they don't like us or don't want to be with us, while ignoring other possible (and probably more likely) explanations. Mind reading demotivates us most strongly from mood-boosting activities that involve social connections with others.

Can you think of an example of mind reading from your own life? Write it down here:

_____

_____

"Should" Statements

When we're depressed, we often think in terms of "should" statements. Thoughts like *I should go to the gym more often*; *I should give my friend a call*; or *I should mow the lawn* all suggest that these activities are moral imperatives—you absolutely *must* do them, and if you don't, you're a failure, a loser, or a bad person. "Should" statements rob us of our motivation by turning our activities into onerous tasks—things that *must* or *ought* to be done, rather than activities that we may enjoy or benefit from. Most people really don't like being told what they "should" do—in fact, it often makes them want to do the exact opposite! And that's true even if we are telling ourselves what we "should" do. It's a real motivation buster!

Can you think of an example of a "should" statement from your own life? Write it down here:

_____

_____

Emotional Reasoning

Emotional reasoning is the faulty belief that if something *feels* true it must *be* true. For example, when you're depressed you may assume that if you *feel* too tired to do anything, that must mean that you *are* too tired to do anything. This is almost always simply not true. We can do many things even when feeling very tired—and as we've seen, we tend to feel less tired once we get rolling!

Try this experiment. Start by rating how tired you are right now and how much energy you have on a scale from 1 to 10. Now put down this book and stand up. Next, do a little gentle stretching. Roll your shoulders and stand on your toes. Do it a few times. You might also bend your knees. Can you take a small jump, and maybe a second one—or even just walk around the room? Touch your toes. Now rate how tired you are and your level of energy. Was there a change?

Even if your energy didn't change, you've just proven to yourself that feeling tired does *not* mean that you can't do anything. You may even be starting to feel a bit less tired.

Can you think of an example of emotional reasoning from your own life? Write it down here:

_____

_____

What About You?

It's now time for you to identify some of your motivation-busting thoughts. The easiest way to do this is to think of a specific mood-boosting activity that you had planned and then either avoided or had trouble getting motivated for. Read Maya's example, and then ask yourself, *What was going through my mind that made it so hard for me to get started?* Next, write these thoughts down—as many as you can remember—below.

Maya's mood-boosting activity: *Playing board games with my kids on Thursday night*

Thoughts running through Maya's head:

It won't be much fun.

My kids don't enjoy playing games with me.

I'm too tired for this.

My mood-boosting activity _____

Thoughts running through my head:

_____

_____

_____

_____

_____

Now, look at the thoughts you identified and see if they fit into a thinking trap. Use the *Identifying Thinking Traps* worksheet below. Again, we've filled in a few of Maya's responses as examples. Keep in mind that you can be caught in more than one thinking trap at a time. Don't worry if you are not sure which thinking trap is right for your thoughts, or if your thoughts don't fit neatly into one of the thinking traps we focused on. What matters is that you start noticing the thoughts that go with your depression and zap your motivation.

Identifying Thinking Traps (Fortune-telling, catastrophizing, mind reading, "should" statements, emotional reasoning)	
Motivation-busting thought	**Thinking trap**
It won't be much fun.	Fortune-telling
My kids don't enjoy playing games with me.	Mind-reading
I'm too tired for this.	Emotional reasoning

Challenge Your Motivation-Busting Thoughts and Develop Motivation-Boosting Thoughts

When we are caught in a thinking trap we tend to believe our thoughts—they just "feel" true. However, when we stop and look at these thoughts more closely, we often discover that not only are they unhelpful for us, but they're also inaccurate or unbalanced in subtle but important ways. We're going to guide you through a few questions that will help you evaluate your demotivating thinking patterns and develop some motivation-boosting thoughts.

Does This Thought Help Get Me Motivated?

All else being equal, you want your thoughts to be helpful to you. If a thought brings you down or demotivates you from engaging in mood-boosting activities, then it's probably not very helpful. As we saw earlier, "should" statements like *I should go to the gym more often* are examples of thoughts that undermine motivation.

So how could you make this thought more helpful? What if you try to be kind and gentle to yourself, and turn the "should" statement into a suggestion. For example, say to yourself, *I'll probably feel a lot better if I go to the gym more often.* Do you see the difference? The "should" statement is a threat—*Do it or else!* The alternative is kinder and creates a positive incentive that is much more motivating.

What's the Evidence?

Motivation-busting thoughts are very much like habits—we get accustomed to having them, and it doesn't occur to us to question their accuracy. But it can be very helpful to step back and examine the evidence for these thoughts. You'll want to consider the evidence both for *and* against your thoughts. One really good way to do this is to imagine putting your thoughts on trial in a court of law. What would be the evidence in favor of your thoughts? What would be the evidence against your thoughts? If a judge were weighing the evidence, what would the verdict be?

It can often be particularly hard to think of the evidence against your thoughts. Try to ask yourself, *What evidence would a good friend or family member think of if they knew I was thinking this way?* Also, try this question: *Is there any evidence against my motivation-busting thoughts that I am ignoring—even small pieces of evidence?*

Maya decided to put the thoughts *It won't be much fun* and *The kids don't enjoy playing games with me* on trial. She remembered that the last time she played games with her kids, everyone had a really good time, and her children had been asking to play with her again. She could not actually remember a specific time when they had not enjoyed playing games together. Maya smiled as she recognized that she didn't have much evidence for her thoughts. She decided that the thought *It's pretty likely that the kids will want to play games with me and that we'll have a good time together* was more balanced and fit better with the evidence. Maya wrote it down and even said it to herself a few times. To her surprise, she began to feel much more motivated to play board games with her children.

What Else Could It Be?

It's always useful to ask yourself whether there is another way to look at a situation or whether there may be another explanation. This is particularly important for thinking traps like mind reading. So, for example, rather than jumping to the conclusion that a friend dislikes you because they don't return a text message right away, ask yourself, *What else could it be?* Maybe your friend's phone was silenced or misplaced. Maybe your friend was in an all-day meeting. Maybe your friend was sick.

Another way to look for alternative explanations is to ask yourself what a good friend would tell you if they knew you were having these thoughts—or what you would tell a good friend who was having them.

Reminding yourself that there may be alternate explanations can help with your motivation to connect with others. By the way, you'll probably be surprised how often these other explanations turn out to be true!

Your Turn

We want you to get a feel for what it's like to challenge your motivation-busting thoughts and transform them into motivation-boosting thoughts. You can use the questions that follow to guide you through this process.

Start by identifying a recent mood-boosting activity where you felt really unmotivated, or perhaps a mood-boosting activity you avoided (or wanted to avoid) because you were too tired or just couldn't find the motivation to do it.

My low-motivation activity/situation:

_____

Next, write down a motivation-busting thought that was going through your mind at the time.

_____

Write down any thinking trap(s) that may capture this thought.

_____

Now challenge your thought by asking yourself the following questions:

Is this thought helpful?

_____

What evidence supports this thought?

_____

What evidence challenges this thought?

_____

Is there another way of looking at this situation?

_____

Finally, see if you can come up with a different thought that is more helpful, more balanced—and more motivating. Try to think of a thought that would be kinder and more compassionate toward yourself.

_____

_____

_____

Challenging and transforming our thoughts can be a difficult skill to learn. This may have been the first time you tried to develop more helpful, balanced thinking. Keep at it. It will get easier with practice.

"Stop" and "Go" Thoughts

Getting started with a behavioral activation plan is often the hardest part. When we're depressed, we tend to have a lot of thoughts that discourage us from taking action and tempt us to cancel or avoid our mood-boosting activities. We call these "stop" thoughts. In this section we're going to help you develop a list of thoughts that will do just the opposite—give you a push to start your behavioral activation plans. We call these "go" thoughts.

Below are some "go" thoughts that have helped our clients over the years get started with behavioral activation. We've divided them into two categories: (1) thoughts that can help motivate you to get going on your behavioral activation plans, and (2) thoughts that can help you manage the depressing thoughts and feelings that can zap your motivation.

Thoughts to help you get going:

- *I have a plan.*

- *Do the first step of my plan.*

- *Try my plan for five minutes.*

- *Focus on the task.*

- *It doesn't have to be perfect.*

- *One step at a time.*

- *What's the next thing?*

- *Even if I'm upset, I can follow my plan.*

- *I can do it.*

- *I know what to do.*

- _____

- _____

Thoughts to help you manage your motivation-busting thoughts and feelings:

- *I don't have to listen to negative thoughts.*

- *It's just my depression saying I won't like it—I'll try it.*

- *Just because I'm depressed doesn't mean I have to stay home.*

- *I made a plan, so I'll stick to it; I won't second guess myself.*

- *I care about my family and myself—that means engaging in life even if I don't feel like it.*

- *Remember my core values.*

- *Feeling too tired doesn't mean that I am too tired.*

- _____

- _____

Maya looked at this list of "go" thoughts. She really liked: *It's just my depression saying I won't like it—I'll try it.* She thought it would be helpful to remember this when she wanted to contact old friends.

Look back at these "go" thoughts, and circle any that stand out to you and that you could use to jump-start your motivation. Try asking yourself these questions:

- What thoughts would I suggest to a friend (think of a specific person) to boost their motivation if they were in this situation and had this thought?

- How would this friend boost my motivation?

- How have I handled similar situations in the past?

- What has helped me get going?

Use the blank lines to add these additional thoughts to your list of "go" thoughts.

Use Core Values to Develop "Go" Thoughts

Remembering your core values can help you develop your own "go" thoughts. If you're having trouble getting motivated for a particular activity, reflect on why this activity may be important to you. Think about the core values you identified in chapter 5—are any of them relevant to this activity? Ask yourself, *If I acted according to my core values, what would I say to myself?* or *What could I say to myself to remind myself of my core values?*

Maya and Nina explored why starting to work on her mother's estate was important to her. Maya identified the core value of being financially responsible to herself and her family. Her "go" thoughts were "This is important to me" and "I want to be a financially responsible person." Maya felt more motivated to work on her mother's estate once she identified the related core values—though she still did not particularly enjoy it.

Your Turn

Let's practice developing and using "go" thoughts for specific situations. Again, start by identifying a mood-boosting activity that you're having difficulty getting motivated to do. It could be the same one you chose in the previous section or a different one. Write it down here:

_____

On the blank lines, list some "go" thoughts that might help you get going on this mood-boosting activity. You can use "go" thoughts from the list of examples we gave you earlier, including any you may have come up with yourself. You can also add any "go" thoughts related to your core values—what you would say to yourself if you were acting on what really matters to you.

_____

_____

_____

_____

_____

From this list of "go" thoughts, select two or three that will really help you get going with your behavioral activation plan. Write them down on sticky notes and put them someplace where you'll see them regularly (for example, on your bathroom mirror or your computer screen). Being reminded of your "go" thoughts will help keep you motivated and on track. You may even find it helpful to think of a shorthand statement that captures your "go" thoughts. Ed's shorthand "go" thought was *Just do it!*

Practice Makes...Better

You probably can't eliminate thoughts that undermine your motivation—and ironically, trying not to think certain thoughts makes us think about them even more! However, the more you challenge your thinking traps, the weaker and less believable they will become. Conversely, the more you practice the thoughts that get and keep you motivated—your helpful, balanced thoughts and your "go" thoughts—the more likely you'll be to listen to them and act on them.

Below is a list of different ways you can strengthen both your helpful, balanced thinking and your "go" thoughts.

- Regularly review your motivation-boosting thoughts. Set a specific time to review them each day. Write them down, put them in your smartphone, set a timer to remind yourself to look at them. Say your "go" thoughts out loud, standing straight with your shoulders back. (You may feel a bit silly doing this, but try it—it works!)

- Review your "go" thoughts when it's time to start a mood-boosting activity.

- Review the evidence against your thinking traps—it's easy to forget.

- Conduct little experiments to test your thinking traps. For example, when you have the thought *I'm too tired*, notice what happens to your energy level and motivation when you go ahead and engage in an activity anyway. As another example, keep track of how frequently things turn out as horribly as you thought they would. You may be surprised at how bad you are at predicting the future!

- Use imaginal rehearsal. Choose a mood-boosting activity, and imagine it's time to do the activity. First, answer back to any thinking traps with evidence. Then, repeat your "go" thoughts in your mind—really hear them. Say them out loud to yourself a few times. Now, imagine yourself doing the activity. At the end of the activity, imagine feeling good. Repeat this whole sequence in your imagination another two times.

What's Next?

In this chapter we've focused on thoughts—how we can challenge mood- and motivation-busting thinking patterns and develop more helpful, motivation-boosting thoughts.

What ideas from this chapter would you like to try in your own life?

_____

What could be motivating for you next week?

_____

If you did a behavioral activation activity last week, what helped you get and stay motivated?

_____

Would you like to make a plan to use a motivation-boosting-strategy?

_____

Look at this illustration for a summary of how you can use your thoughts to boost your motivation.

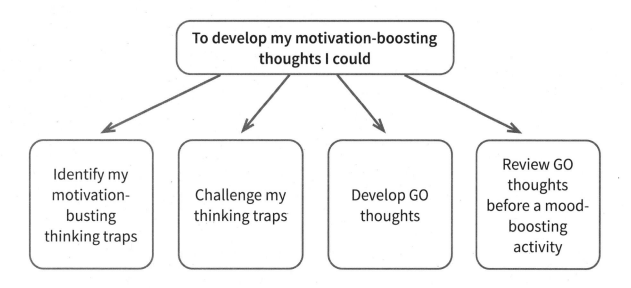

Figure 9.2: Develop Motivation-Boosting Thoughts

We know it's not easy to get going and stay going when you're depressed. Making changes takes courage and determination. Don't give up! You're worth the effort.

In the next chapter we're going to introduce you to a new set of skills based on mindfulness that you can use to weaken the grip of depression's motivation-busting thoughts and feelings. We've taught these skills to hundreds of clients who have found them to be very helpful. We think you will too.

CHAPTER 10

Use Mindfulness to Deal with Motivation-Busting Thoughts and Feelings

Depression undermines our motivation and discourages us from doing the very things that would help us feel better. It can be persistent. No matter how much progress you've made in your behavioral activation work, you will probably continue to some have negative, motivation-busting thoughts and feelings from time to time. You may be wondering *Is there anything else I can do?* And there is—a very practical tool known as *mindfulness*.

What Is Mindfulness and How Can It Help?

Put simply, mindfulness involves deliberately and purposefully paying attention to the thoughts, feelings, and senses that we are experiencing in the present moment. Very importantly, it involves doing so with an attitude of openness and curiosity—free of judgment, evaluation, or analysis (Kabat-Zinn 1990). As we cultivate mindfulness, we learn to observe our here-and-now experiences with a greater degree of acceptance and allow them to run their course without making efforts to resist, change, or react to them in any way. Ironically, the more we accept our negative thoughts and feelings and the less we fight them, the weaker they become.

When we're depressed, negative thoughts like *There's no point in doing anything* or *I'm a complete loser* seem like self-evident truths that spin around and around in our brains. We feel sad, lethargic, and tired—and it can be hard to imagine ever feeling anything different. Mindfulness helps us step back and get some distance from our negative thoughts and feelings, allowing us to simply observe them in much the same way a curious scientist might observe an interesting scientific phenomenon. When we step back from our negative, demotivating thoughts and feelings—and this is particularly important in the context of behavioral activation—we discover that we don't have to react or give in to them, but that we are free to respond to situations on the basis of our values and priorities. As a result, those thoughts and feelings begin to lose their power to control our actions.

Try a Simple Mindfulness Exercise

We'd like to introduce you to mindfulness firsthand. We'll keep it really simple and brief—maybe five to ten minutes at the most—just to give you a little taste of what being mindful is like.

To start, find a quiet place with as few distractions as possible. You'll want to set your phone to "do not disturb." Sit in a comfortable chair with your feet on the floor and your hands supported on your chair or your lap.

Once you've settled in, close your eyes if you're comfortable doing so, or if not, fix your eyes on a spot on the floor. Start by taking in a slow, deep breath through your nose, holding it for a moment, then slowly exhaling through your mouth. Then do it again.

Continue to breathe normally while focusing your attention on your breath. Notice the sensations associated with the air flowing through your nostrils and nasal passages, moving down into your lungs and then back up through your nose again. Pay attention to the movement of your body as you inhale and exhale. Observe the difference in the temperature of the air as it flows in and flows out. Pay close attention to your breath.

Inevitably, despite trying to focus on your breath, your mind will wander. You will catch yourself having a variety of thoughts (for example, *What am I having for dinner tonight?* or *This is silly!* or *Why is that new guy at work being so mean to me?*). You may also become aware of other feelings or sensations (for example, noticing your heart beating, hearing street noises). When this happens (and believe us, it will!), you can take a moment to note whatever thoughts, feelings, or sensations your mind has brought into your awareness—remember, no self-judgment or criticism. Then gently let them go and draw your attention back to your breath. Do this over and over—as often as necessary. It's actually a very important part of the exercise because it reinforces your ability to let go of your thoughts and feelings—to acknowledge them as they pass through your mind, without getting caught up or enmeshed in them.

After doing this for a few minutes, you can gently open your eyes again (if you had them closed). Feel free to give yourself a stretch. Congratulations! You've just completed a simple mindfulness exercise.

Let's take a moment to debrief. Here are a few questions you can ask yourself. We've left space for you to write down your reflections.

What sensations did you notice while doing your breathing?

_____

_____

What did you notice when you tried to focus on your breath?

_____

_____

What was it like to try and acknowledge these thoughts and feelings and then let them go and draw your attention back to your breath?

_____

_____

If you had any other observations, add them here:

_____

_____

Everyone's experience of mindfulness is unique and there is no "right" or "wrong" way to respond. However, we hope that this brief exercise gave you some sense of what it's like to simply observe your here-and-now experience—your breath, of course, but also the additional thoughts and feelings you had—without judging, analyzing, or reacting to them in any way.

You might be wondering *How is this exercise related to my depression?* Well, just as you started noticing your breath, your thoughts, your feelings, and your sensations without reacting to them, you can also learn to observe your negative feelings and thoughts without reacting to them. It's kind of like surfing. If you think of your negative, demotivating thoughts and feelings as a big wave on the ocean, mindfulness is like surfing that wave. Rather than resisting it, ignoring it, or trying to escape it, you can learn to just ride it out.

Using HUMP and the 3 Ns

We want to introduce you to a very practical tool we've developed for applying mindfulness in your everyday life: HUMP and the 3 Ns. We've shared it with many of our clients over the years—including Ed and Maya. We think you will find it helpful. You can use it to remind yourself how to step back from your mood- and motivation-busting thoughts and feelings and respond to them in a way that gives them as little power over you as possible.

Tell Yourself the Truth about Your Negative Thoughts and Feelings—HUMP

We all have thoughts and feelings—but we also react to our thoughts and feelings. For example, Ed believed that his anxiety about attending a retraining class meant that he was a loser—and this made him want to quit the class. When Maya had the thought *I will never get better*, she assumed it must be true—and of course felt even worse. What we tell ourselves about our own thoughts and feelings can have a significant impact on how they affect us and can influence how we react to them. In this section we'll focus on four key truths about your negative thoughts and feelings. Then we'll consider the implications of these truths for how you can respond to your thoughts and feelings.

H—*They're Harmless*

The first thing you need to know about your depressive, motivation-busting thoughts and feelings is that they are completely harmless. They are, after all, just thoughts and feelings. While they may be unpleasant and even painful at times, they are not intrinsically dangerous or harmful. Of course, acting on your negative thoughts and feelings can potentially create a great deal of trouble. Take Ed's anxious feelings about starting a retraining course as an example. If Ed had acted on his anxious feelings, he would have stopped attending the course—and this would have sabotaged his plans for the future. Using a mindful approach, Ed acknowledged that, while the anxious feelings were unpleasant, they were not harmful or dangerous. He could feel anxious and still make the decision to continue with the class. And he did.

U—They're Useless

The second truth about your motivation-busting depressive thoughts and feelings is that they don't serve any real purpose. They're useless. They don't help you live a better life; they don't protect you from danger; and they don't provide you with any helpful guidance or direction. All they do is demotivate you and, if acted upon, shut you down. Maya, for example, wanted to start meeting with her friends again. She was able to see that the thought *I will never get better* did not help her achieve this goal. It was a useless thought.

We certainly don't mean to suggest that all your thoughts and feelings are useless—because that's most definitely not the case. Under normal circumstances, our thoughts and our emotions can provide important information that helps us navigate the world in a safe, effective, and meaningful way. However, when we're depressed many of our thoughts and feelings are simply a reflection of our depression, and they stop serving us in a useful fashion.

M—They're Meaningless

Not only are motivation-busting thoughts and feelings harmless and useless, they're also meaningless. That is, what they tell us is not necessarily true. For example, Maya's thought *I will never get better* did not actually mean that Maya would never get better. It was just a thought—and *thoughts are not truths*. Similarly, Ed's feeling of lethargy and tiredness in the morning didn't mean that he was unable to get out of bed, or that he couldn't engage in helpful, mood-boosting activities. His tiredness was just a feeling—and *feelings are not facts*.

> *Thoughts Are Not Truths*
>
> *Feelings Are Not Facts*

P—They're Passing

The fourth—and possibly the most important—thing to keep in mind about all your thoughts and feelings is that they are transient, or passing. You've never had a thought or feeling that lasted forever—and you never will! All thoughts and feelings—even very negative and painful ones—come and go on their own if left to run their own course. Ironically, it's only when we try to stop our thoughts and feelings, focus on them, or worry about having them that they hang around.

Negative thoughts and feelings are like the weather. They're always changing—coming and going.

If you were to plot on a graph the trajectory of your negative thoughts and feelings—that is, their intensity over time—you would notice that they build in intensity, reach a peak, and then begin to ease, as illustrated below. Test it out for yourself. Next time you notice yourself getting really upset about something, try to ride it out. Notice how your feelings build, reach a peak, and then start to fade all by themselves.

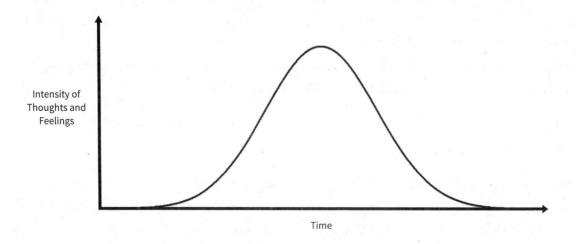

Figure 10.1: The Trajectory of Thoughts and Feelings Over Time

You may have noticed that the shape of the curve above looks a bit like a camel's hump. Use the image of a camel's hump to remind you of HUMP—harmless, useless, meaningless, and passing!

Respond Mindfully to Motivation-Busting Thoughts and Feelings—The 3 Ns

Rather than reacting to your negative thoughts and feelings and getting caught up in the negative cycle of depression, we want to show you how to respond mindfully. When you respond mindfully to your negative thoughts and feelings, they lose their power. There are three steps and they all involve the letter N, so we call them the 3 Ns.

Notice Them

The first step in responding mindfully to your negative thoughts and feelings is to pause and simply *notice* them. This means stepping back and observing your thoughts and feelings. Notice what images or thoughts your mind is presenting to you. Pay attention to the sensations in your body. Again, think of yourself as a scientist—observing your own experience with curiosity and openness. Remember, your thoughts and feeling will come and go just like the weather.

Stepping back and noticing your negative thoughts and feelings is hard at first. However, it's a skill that can be learned by practicing mindfulness on a regular basis.

Name Them

The next step in responding to your motivation-busting thoughts and feelings involves labeling them or giving them a *name*. Research has shown that when we name our negative thoughts and feelings they tend to lose some of their grip on us (Torre and Lieberman 2018).

Since you tend to experience the same old depressive thoughts and feelings over and over again, it makes sense to develop a list—a collection of your "greatest hits," each with its own name.

Some people like to come up with humorous names for their thoughts and feelings. For example, Ed decided to name his demotivating feeling of lethargy "Mr. Blob" since that's how it made him feel—like a blob. Ed also came up with a name for his demotivating thought *What's the point?* Ed called this thought "The Pointless Sisters" after a seventies-era rock group his mother had liked as a teenager. Giving his thoughts and feelings humorous names really helped Ed get a different perspective on them and see them as distinct from himself.

Do Nothing About Them

We've established that your motivation-busting thoughts are harmless, useless, meaningless, and that they're going to pass all by themselves. So what's the best thing to do about them? The answer is…absolutely…*nothing!* What does doing nothing mean? Let's look at some "dos and don'ts" of what it means to do nothing about your motivation-busting thoughts and feelings.

We'll start by looking at the don'ts. First, *don't* try to avoid your negative thoughts and feelings or try to get rid of them in any way. Remember, these thoughts and feelings will come and go all by themselves, with no help from you. In fact, the harder you work at trying to avoid or get rid of them, the longer they will last and the more intense they will become—just the opposite of what you intend.

Second, *don't* let your motivation-busting thoughts or feelings boss you around or tell you how to act. Think of them as bad advice. So, for example, when a lethargic feeling (like Mr. Blob) tells you to sit on the couch for the afternoon—don't do it! Doing what negative thoughts and feelings tell you to do just gives them the oxygen they need to persist and flourish.

Third, *don't* analyze or try to figure out your motivation-busting thoughts and feelings. Asking yourself *Why am I feeling this way?* or *Why am I having this thought?* is unlikely to be all that helpful. It's important to note your sad thoughts and feelings and accept them, but focusing on them and trying to figure out where they come from just gives them more power—more oxygen. Of course there are reasons for our negative thoughts and feelings—they may be related to difficult events in our lives, to how much sleep we've had, to biochemical or hormonal changes, or to many other factors. But focusing on the why rarely helps. In fact, asking why you feel the way you do often implies that you shouldn't be feeling what you're feeling—and telling yourself you shouldn't be feeling what you do feel can only make you feel worse!

So, what are the *dos* in "doing nothing" about your motivation-busting thoughts and feelings? The answer is actually quite simple. Ask yourself, *What would I be doing right now if I weren't having these negative, motivation-busting thoughts or feelings?* Then go ahead and do it! Do whatever it is that you would be doing if you were not having those thoughts or feelings (even though you *are* having them). When you do this, you are acting on your values, not on your negative thoughts and feelings. And this is what it means, in a positive way, to do nothing about them.

> *What would I be doing right now if I were not having this negative,*
> *motivation-busting thought or feeling?*

Ed reflected on what it meant to do nothing about "The Pointless Sisters" when they came for a visit in the morning as he was lying in bed feeling depressed. He asked himself what he would be doing if he were not having the thought *What's the point?* He concluded that he'd be getting up and taking a shower. So that's exactly what he did. Ed noticed his thoughts, but he did not act on them—he did "nothing" about his motivation- and mood-busting thought.

Doing nothing about your negative thoughts and feelings isn't easy. It takes courage and practice. The good news is that it's a skill you can learn, and it gets easier over time. We think you'll be surprised to discover that those thoughts and feelings come and go all by themselves while you're busy engaging in mood-boosting activities.

One last reminder. Using HUMP and the 3 Ns is not about changing or getting rid of your negative, motivation-busting thoughts and feelings. It's a strategy for giving them less and less power over you and depriving them of the fuel they need to continue undermining your motivation and taking you out of the game. The more you practice, the easier it will be.

HUMP and the 3 Ns

My negative thoughts and feelings are:

Harmless

Useless

Meaningless

Passing

Therefore I can:

Notice them

Name them

Do **N**othing about them

What About You?

Are you ready to try HUMP and the 3 Ns on your own mood-busting thoughts and feelings? Let's start with identifying a specific thought or feeling associated with low motivation for you. Write down your motivation-busting thought or feeling here:

_____

Now remind yourself that these demotivating thoughts or feeling are harmless, useless, and meaningless, and that they will pass all by themselves. Sometimes it's helpful to say out loud, "This thought (or this feeling) is harmless, useless, meaningless, and passing."

If you're experiencing this thought or feeling right now, try to step back and observe it as something that is happening to you, rather than as a truth or an unchangeable reality. Don't judge or evaluate it—just *notice* it.

Now let's see if you can come up with a name for this thought or feeling. Remember, Ed called his thought "The Pointless Sisters" and his feeling "Mr. Blob." Write yours here:

_____

Having noticed and named your negative, demotivating thought or feeling, you can now make the choice to do nothing about it. If you're tempted to act on that thought or feeling in some way—don't do it! If you're trying to avoid or get rid of the thought or feeling in some way—don't do it! If you're trying to figure out why you're feeling or thinking that way—don't do it! Instead, ask yourself, *If I were not having this negative, demotivating thought or feeling, what would I be doing right now?* Write down your answer here:

_____

_____

Now go ahead and do whatever it is that you would be doing. Remember, your demotivating thoughts and feelings are harmless, useless, meaningless, and passing—so you really don't have to let them stop you from taking mood-boosting action. Take a moment to reflect on how different your life could be if you practiced HUMP and the 3 Ns. We hope you'll find this truth liberating and empowering.

What's Next?

In this chapter we've introduced you to the concept of mindfulness and given you a practical mindfulness-based tool—HUMP and the 3 Ns—that you can use to give your negative, motivation-busting thoughts and feelings less power. As you reflect on this chapter, what resonated most strongly with you?

_____

_____

_____

Identify any upcoming situations in which using this approach could be useful, and then write down how you could use HUMP and the 3 Ns in these situations. Take a moment to imagine these situations actually happening, and see yourself using HUMP and the 3 Ns.

_____

_____

_____

_____

_____

We've now covered several powerful strategies for building motivation and dealing with the motivation-busting thoughts and feelings that keep you from doing the kinds of activities that would help you feel better. These are summarized below.

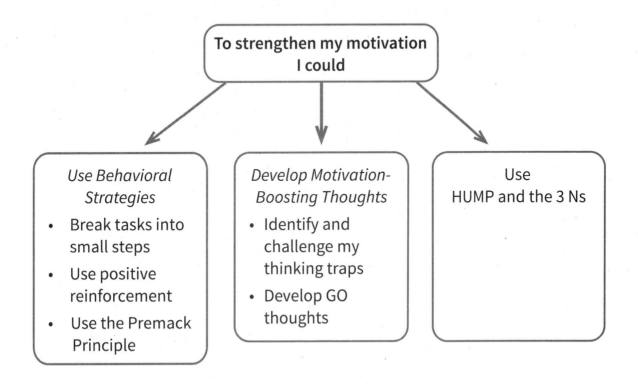

Figure 10.2: Overview of Motivation-Boosting Strategies

Which would you like to try this coming week?

_____

_____

_____

_____

Now congratulate yourself for the important steps you've been taking toward pushing back on your depression and building a better life for yourself.

In the next chapter we'll focus on a number of strategies for maintaining the gains that you've made in creating a depression-resistant life. Then, in the final chapter, we'll explore ways of moving beyond your depression and bringing true happiness and well-being into your life.

PART FOUR

Maintain Your Gains... and Beyond

CHAPTER 11

Keep Your Depression-Resistant Life Going

To maintain a depression-resistant life, it's important to develop healthy routines. Though they will differ from person to person, healthy routines generally involve engaging in both mood-boosting behaviors *and* activities related to self-care on a regular basis. Let's take a closer look at what it means to take care of yourself—and how you can make self-care part of a routine that promotes emotional stability and psychological resilience.

Follow a Healthy Diet

Maintaining good physical health is one of the keys to a happy, fulfilling, depression-resistant life. We've already discussed the impact that exercise and physical activity can have on your mood, and your mental health in general. Maintaining a regular routine of physical activity is one of the most effective ways of keeping depression at bay and maximizing the enjoyment of your life.

What we eat is a key factor in good health—but did you know that it can also affect the likelihood of our becoming depressed (Li et al. 2017)? Eating plenty of fresh fruit and vegetables, whole grains, fish, and other natural foods, while minimizing your consumption of sweets, highly processed foods, and red meats, is not only healthy for you physically, but it can also decrease your chances of becoming depressed and keep you psychologically resilient.

A depression-resistant diet is virtually identical to the US and Canada food guidelines. Take a look at the guidelines and see if you want to make any changes to your diet. You can find the Canadian guidelines at: https://food-guide.canada.ca/en/ and the US guidelines at: https://www.fao.org/nutrition/education/food-dietary-guidelines/regions/countries/united-states-of-america/en/. Even small changes to your diet can make a big difference when it comes to maintaining good mental health.

Get Enough Good Sleep

Sleep is a key factor in a depression-resistant lifestyle. Depression often negatively affects our sleep. But it works the other way too—poor sleep or insufficient sleep can contribute to low mood and make us more vulnerable to slipping back into depression. Although it can vary from person to person, experts agree that most adults need seven to nine hours of sleep per night (Hirshkowitz et al. 2015).

An important caveat: Sleeping difficulties can be very complex and often require comprehensive assessment and specialized treatment. If you are consistently having difficulty sleeping and/or you consistently feel sleepy and unrested, we encourage you to speak to a health professional with expertise in sleep problems.

Psychologists have identified a number of sleep-boosting steps you can take to maximize the likelihood of regularly getting a good night's rest (Manber and Carney 2015). Take a look at the suggestions below and see which might be helpful for you.

Establish Regular Sleep-Wake Routines

Try to go to bed at approximately the same time every night, and then get up at about the same time every morning. Our bodies—and our brains—like routines, and we tend to sleep better when we've established a regular sleep-wake pattern. You want to train your body's biological clock.

Limit Your Naps

Naps can be enjoyable and in many cultures, people nap regularly. However, if you nap too long—or too late in the day—you'll risk disrupting the regular sleep-wake routine that you're trying to establish. If you want to nap, try to do so in the early afternoon for a maximum of thirty minutes. That way you'll be tired at night and ready to sleep.

Be Careful About Caffeine and Alcohol

Caffeine can be the kiss of death for a good night's sleep. Many different foods and drinks contain caffeine—coffee, tea, hot chocolate, many sodas and energy drinks and chocolate bars. If you're having trouble sleeping, experiment with cutting out caffeine within several hours of bedtime—or even eliminating it completely. Some people can have caffeine right before they go to bed and it never affects their sleep. In some cultures, people regularly drink coffee at night. However, other people need up to ten hours for caffeine to completely leave their body. I (Nina) unfortunately am definitely a "coffee keeps me up" person. Every so often, usually when I am out with friends, I order a cappuccino—and then at 3:00 a.m. I promise myself I will never have another cup of coffee before bed! What about you? How do you think caffeine affects you?

What about alcohol? Drinking alcohol before you go to bed can make you feel sleepy and may even help you fall asleep. But alcohol also leads to early waking and to getting a more fragmented, less restful sleep. Try decreasing how much alcohol you drink and see if it makes a difference.

Eat Lightly Before Bedtime

Eating a heavy meal right before bedtime can disrupt your sleep cycle. If you're having trouble sleeping, try eating earlier. A very light snack just before bedtime is fine and may even be helpful.

Develop a Relaxing Bedtime Routine

A relaxing bedtime routine sends a signal to your body that it's time to wind down for the evening. Many people find that spending time on their cell phones and computers makes them feel wired and can make it more difficult to fall asleep. Experiment with turning off your phone an hour or two before you go to sleep. Similarly, vigorous exercise just before bedtime can energize you and make it difficult to fall asleep.

Create a Sleep-Friendly Environment

We tend to rest better in sleep-friendly environments—in rooms that are dark, quiet, and at a comfortable temperature. If there is a lot of noise where you sleep, try masking the sound by using a white-noise machine or a fan. Similarly, if your bedroom has a lot of light, try wearing a sleep mask.

Associate Your Bed with Sleep

You want your body to associate being in bed with sleeping. This means that when you are in bed—sleep and sex, nothing else. No reading, watching TV, or eating in bed. That just weakens the brain's association between your bed and being asleep. Furthermore, if during the night you are lying awake for more than twenty minutes, get out of bed. Do something relaxing and enjoyable (for example, read a book, do crossword puzzles, listen to music) until you start to feel sleepy. Then go back to bed. It's hard to get yourself out of bed in the middle of the night, but it's important to train your brain to associate your bed only with sleeping.

Don't Panic If You Don't Get a Good Night's Sleep

Racing or anxious thoughts can wreak havoc with our sleep. If you are waking up in the middle of the night worrying or upset about a situation in your life, try to take a few deep breaths and then gently remind yourself that the middle of the night is not a good time to solve your problems. Write down your concerns so you can remember them in the morning. Allow yourself to gently put the worry aside. Acknowledge that you're upset and then tell yourself you can deal with the situation in the morning. Now take a few deep breaths. In a gentle compassionate voice tell yourself it's okay to just go back to sleep. You could also listen to a guided relaxation or mindfulness exercise to help redirect your mind.

Many people put a lot of pressure on themselves to fall asleep and to stay asleep. They tell themselves, *I've got to get to sleep right away or else I'm going to have a horrible day tomorrow.* Other people worry: *If I don't get seven hours of sleep tonight, I'll fall apart and get depressed again.* The fact of the matter is that most of us can function quite well on very limited sleep for brief periods of time. Ironically, when we worry about sleeping, it is even *more* difficult to fall asleep and stay asleep. Trust your body to get the sleep it needs and don't worry about not sleeping…then drift off!

What About You?

In this section, you'll find a *Sleep Self-Evaluation* worksheet. Do you remember Eva from chapter 3 who was being sexually harassed at work? When she completed the *Sleep Self-Evaluation* worksheet she realized she had started eating before bed as a way to comfort herself, and often went to bed with an excessively full stomach. Because she wasn't sleeping well she was chronically tired and had increased how much coffee she drank during the day. She had even started having a cup of coffee at 4:00 p.m. She realized that she spent the time just before bed thinking over the day's events and telling her partner how much she hated her boss and how trapped she felt. She would go to bed highly agitated. Nina and Eva problem-solved around how to develop a better pre-bedtime routine. She decided to reduce her snacking before bed, cut out her afternoon coffee, set a time to think about the day's events that was well before bedtime, and engage in relaxing, soothing activities before bed. While Eva's sleep wasn't perfect, these changes helped to generally improve her sleep.

It's now time for you to evaluate your sleep. First, take a look at the *Sleep Self-Evaluation* worksheet and see how you are doing. Then, write down what you would like to try doing differently.

Sleep Self-Evaluation		
Sleep booster	**How am I doing?**	**What I would like to try doing differently**
Follow regular sleep-wake routines		
Limit naps to midday and no more than a half hour		
Limit caffeine		

Sleep booster	How am I doing?	What I would like to try doing differently
Be careful with the amount of alcohol you drink		
Eat lightly before bedtime		
Develop a relaxing bedtime routine. Try turning off your cell phone before bed.		
Create a sleep-friendly environment		
Associate bed with sleep—no eating, reading, or watching TV		
Get out of bed after twenty minutes of not sleeping; wait to go back to bed until you are sleepy again		

Take a look at your sleep evaluation worksheet, choose one or two changes that you think might make the biggest difference to your sleep, and commit to making the changes. Try the new routines for a week, then check to see if they have made a difference to your sleep.

Establishing healthy sleep habits and taking care of yourself by staying physically active and maintaining healthy eating patterns are an important foundation for reducing the risk of becoming depressed again. They are also important factors in creating a happy, good life. We hope you'll make them part of your life.

Get Ahead of Your Depression: Anticipate and Plan for High-Risk Situations

In this section, we're going to look at two strategies that will help you keep depression from getting a toehold in your life again. The first involves dealing with high-risk situations.

For each of us there are a variety of circumstances—for example, stressors, life changes, conflicts, triggers, difficulties—that have the potential to send us back into the old spiral of depression. We call these "high-risk situations." Often, these high-risk situations disrupt our routines, and we stop engaging in the activities that maintain a positive mood. As our mood drops, we start to have less energy and less motivation. If this continues over a long enough period of time, we may feel down and even get depressed again.

It can be very helpful to identify your particular high-risk situations, and then to create an action plan for coping with them effectively should they arise.

Identify Your High-Risk Situations

To identify your high-risk situations, look back to when you've had setbacks in your mood. What was going on in your life at those times—or maybe just before—that may have contributed to the development of your low mood? Then, see if you can identify how these situations affected your behavior—and in particular, how they affected your engagement in activities you enjoy.

When Maya reflected on these questions, she realized that she often felt down and overwhelmed at report-card time. She realized that she would stop exercising, stay up late to get her work done, and see her friends less. The other time she felt more vulnerable to depression was following days or events that reminded her of her mother's death—like her mother's birthday and Mother's Day. The sadness she experienced on those days often seemed to trigger a deeper depression.

High-risk situations are not always stressful or unhappy times. Ed discovered that during the holiday season—which he generally enjoyed—he got out of the habit of engaging in many of his mastery and achievement activities. He also ate more than usual and engaged in less physical activity. This was often the start of a decline in his mood that resulted in an early-January depression.

What are your high-risk situations? Take a moment to reflect on the situations that you think may put you at risk for setbacks in your mood—and write them down here:

_____

_____

_____

Plan Effective Coping Strategies

Once you've identified your high-risk situations, you can start developing a plan for coping with them. You'll want to lean on three key strategies we've covered in this workbook: behavioral activation; problem solving; and mindfulness-based strategies such as HUMP and the 3 Ns.

It's particularly important to have a few go-to mood-boosting activities that are at the ready for those times when we encounter a high-risk situation. You'll want to focus on activities that reliably boost your mood. Just a reminder: make sure that they are specific and doable, and can be part of your routine. Then plan the first step.

Ed's go-to behavioral activation plan for dealing with his postholiday slump was attending his exercise classes on a regular basis both during and after the holidays.

You'll also want to use your problem-solving skills to face your problems and see how you can make them even a little bit easier. And then use HUMP and the 3 Ns to manage your feelings.

Maya started with problem solving how to make report-card writing easier. She decided to start working on her report cards a bit earlier than she had in the past and to spend a maximum of two hours a night. She also decided to simplify mealtime, maybe even freeze some meals so she wouldn't have to spend time cooking. She also made sure to plan some mood-boosting activities during that time. She decided to prioritize walking at lunchtime with a colleague. With these plans in place, Maya felt more confident about her ability to get her report cards done without feeling as overwhelmed as she had in the past.

When Maya thought about her feelings in relation to her mother, she thought that using HUMP and the 3 Ns would be helpful. She accepted her sad feelings as normal and realized they would pass. As Maya planned for Mother's Day, she rehearsed the 3 Ns she had learned—noticing her feelings of sadness, naming them, and then doing nothing about them. She asked herself what she would be doing if she were not feeling so sad. She decided that she would honor her mother by placing flowers at her grave. With this plan in place, Maya felt better about facing the days that reminded her of her mother, despite the sadness she would inevitably experience.

What About You?

Now it's time for you to plan your own coping strategies. Choose one of the high-risk situations you identified, and write it here:

_____

_____

_____

Behavioral activation plan: What are some go-to mood-boosting activities I can plan to engage in when facing this situation? (Remember you want a plan that is specific and doable, and can be part of your routine.)

_____

_____

_____

Problem-solving plan: Is there anything I could do that would make this situation even a little easier? What could I do about this situation that could help me cope more effectively?

_____

_____

_____

Mindfulness plan: Can I accept my feelings as harmless, useless, meaningless, and passing? What would it mean to "do nothing" in this situation?

_____

_____

_____

You can repeat this process for as many other high-risk situations as you've been able to identify.

Get Ahead of Your Depression: Monitor Your Progress and Respond to Early Warning Signs

Getting depressed again tends to happen slowly. It's often such a gradual decline in mood that we may not even notice it until we're caught in depression. To prevent depression from sneaking back in again, it's helpful to keep an eye on how we're doing. By monitoring our progress, we can catch any changes in our lives that suggest we're getting off track—we call these "early warning signs"—and then take get-back-on-track action to start feeling better.

Use Self-Monitoring

Socrates famously said, "The unexamined life is not worth living." While we wouldn't necessarily go that far, we _are_ big fans of self-monitoring—and we'd certainly encourage you to get into the habit of maintaining some kind of record of your mood over time. It may be as simple as using a 10-point scale to rate and record your mood on a regular basis. This enables you to see if your mood has gone down over time and gives you the chance to take steps toward getting back on track. Some people like to track their moods and other variables more systematically. You can keep a journal, download a mood-monitoring app, or use this _Self-Monitoring Rating Scales_ worksheet.

Self-Monitoring Rating Scales 1 (very poor) to 10 (very good)						
Day	Mood	Energy	Sleep	Nutrition	Mood-boosting activity	Overall
Monday						
Tuesday						
Wednesday						
Thursday						
Friday						
Saturday						
Sunday						

One final thought: Don't overdo the self-monitoring. Too much self-focused attention is not helpful—and in fact is associated with negative feelings (Ingram 1990). You just want to monitor enough so that you catch any decreases in your mood that occur over a period of time. We all have bad days and bad weeks. A bad month, however, should probably get your attention. If you are experiencing a tough time in your life, it's normal to feel sad and upset. That doesn't necessarily mean you are getting depressed again. Remember, tough times won't last forever.

Identify Your Early Warning Signs

One big advantage of self-monitoring is that it can help you identify your own early warning signs. Sometimes changes in mood—more frequent feelings of sadness, irritability, stress, anxiety, or low motivation, among others—can be signs that you are feeling somewhat more down. Similarly, things like spending more time alone, withdrawing from activities you usually enjoy, sleeping more than usual, exercising less frequently, drinking more alcohol, eating more (or less) than usual, procrastinating more, or leaving tasks undone can all signal that you're starting to get off track.

Take a moment to reflect on your own early warning signs. What kinds of things may signal that you are beginning to lose ground? We've provided space for three but feel free to come up with as many as possible.

1. _____

2. _____

3. _____

Get Back on Track

An early warning sign is similar to a car's check engine light. It signals that something's not quite right and that it's time to take action to fix it and keep things from getting any worse. In the case of the check engine light, it usually means you need to add oil. Early warning signs for depression also mean that you need to add oil to your life—just a different kind! Taking mood-boosting action—like adding oil—doesn't have to be all that difficult. You'll want to get a behavioral activation plan going again, problem solve your difficulties, and remember HUMP and the 3 Ns.

Begin by getting a new behavioral activation plan started. If you've stopped exercising regularly, maybe it's time to get that going again. If you've found yourself disengaging from people, then why not send out a text or two? Perhaps you can incorporate activities that give you pleasure or add some mastery and accomplishment activities. If you're avoiding problems, why not make a commitment to face them? If you lack motivation, think about using one of the motivation-boosting strategies you read about earlier. Do whatever it takes to get that positive mood-activity cycle up and running again!

Developing a get-back-on-track action plan is a lot like the mood-boosting action plans we discussed earlier in this workbook. Use this *Get Back on Track* worksheet to get started.

Action Plan: Get Back on Track				
What I'll do	Is my plan...	My first step	Obstacles I may encounter	How I'll handle these obstacles
	☐ specific? ☐ doable? ☐ part of my routine?			
	☐ specific? ☐ doable? ☐ part of my routine?			
	☐ specific? ☐ doable? ☐ part of my routine?			
	☐ specific? ☐ doable? ☐ part of my routine?			

And remember HUMP and the 3 Ns. Chances are if you're feeling a bit more down, you've also been facing some challenges. Taking a mindful approach would mean noticing the painful thoughts and feelings, accepting the difficult events, and letting yourself know it's okay to be upset. It also means reminding yourself that your feelings will pass, that they are not dangerous, and that you can make the decision to act according to your values and desires rather than reacting to your feelings.

What About Therapy and Medication?

For many people, following the behavioral activation steps in this workbook will be enough to make and maintain significant improvements in their mood. However, some people may require more help. Seeing a psychotherapist can be very beneficial. It's hard to start and keep up a behavioral activation plan on your own, and having someone to guide you along can make a big difference.

For other people, antidepressant medication can be an important component of treatment for depression. We've had clients who felt more energized and motivated after taking antidepressant medication, and better able to get started and keep going with their behavioral activation plans. If you're thinking about medication, it's important to consult a qualified health professional.

What's Next

In this chapter we've provided you with tools for keeping your depression-resistant life going. Take a moment to think about what you want to take from this chapter. What did you learn that might help you maintain your depression-resistant life?

_____

_____

_____

_____

How can you bring what was meaningful to you in the chapter into your own life? Would you like to make a plan?

_____

_____

_____

_____

_____

In the next and final chapter, before saying good-bye, we're going to look at strategies for moving beyond depression into a life of true happiness and well-being. We think it's a good way to end.

CHAPTER 12

Cultivate Happiness and Well-Being

Most of us want more than just a life that's free of depression. We also want to experience true happiness—not merely the transient pleasure of a good meal or a fun night out (as nice as these types of experiences can be), but deep and sustained feelings of well-being. As we have seen throughout this book, using behavioral activation to develop routines of values-based, mood-boosting behavior constitutes a big step toward creating this kind of happy life.

But there is another piece to the happiness puzzle. It involves qualities that extend beyond the realm of mood-boosting—personal qualities like gratitude and compassion. When we bring these qualities into our life, we develop resilience and the inner strength to better manage life's difficulties.

Notice Your Personal Strengths

Many of us—especially when we're prone to depression—tend to focus on our failures and dwell on our personal shortcomings and weaknesses. We often ignore or minimize the times when we've shown strength and resilience in the face of difficulties, but noticing these experiences is actually very important. Having a clear sense of how we have shown strength and resilience in the face of difficulties gives us confidence in our own ability to handle whatever life throws at us. We develop an attitude of "This may be hard, but I will be able to manage."

We're going to guide you through some self-reflections to help you recognize any personal strengths you may be overlooking.

Think about the areas of your life that are going well. Friendships? Family relationships? Work projects? Hobbies or interests? Have you been able to overcome difficulties in these areas? Work through conflict? Maintain a routine? Keep to a schedule? These types of successes don't happen by accident. They say something about your personal strengths.

When Maya reflected on the areas in her life that were going well, she acknowledged that, despite her depression, she had been able to get to work on time every day. Her classes were always prepared, and she had kept teaching and participated in all school activities. She began to see that this took care, perseverance, and organization—it didn't happen by magic.

Take a moment to identify some areas that are going well for you—big or small. What do they say about you in terms of your personal strengths? Write them down here:

_____

_____

_____

_____

_____

Think about the difficulties you got through. Can you think of a challenging time in your life that you managed to get through? Maybe it was a time in your life that involved a lot of change—a move, a new baby, a new relationship, a new job. Maybe you or a loved one experienced a serious illness. Maybe it was a significant loss or a failure—in a relationship, at work, or at school. Maybe a serious personal conflict. Whatever it was, you made it through. Surviving difficult times takes resilience and grit.

Maya thought about the fact that she had managed to survive a divorce and having her boyfriend cheat on her. She recognized that her ability to come through these times—as hard as they were—reflected courage and inner strength.

What difficulties have you survived?

_____

_____

_____

What does this say about you?

_____

_____

_____

Think about your caring relationships. Caring relationships require commitment, an ability to put aside your own needs and to act unselfishly.

Despite his depression, Ed still found time to play with Alex. He was able to acknowledge that this reflected personal strengths of kindness, gentleness, and fatherly love.

Take a moment to consider the caring relationships that you have—with a person or even a pet. What does this relationship say about you as a person? Write down your thoughts here:

_____

_____

_____

Notice when you act on your values. Is there an area in your life where you are acting according to your values—even when it's not immediately enjoyable? These activities often suggest important underlying strengths.

Despite wanting to avoid everything related to her mother's estate taxes, Maya eventually got them taken care of. She was able to recognize that she had found the strength to do something very difficult when it was important to her.

Is there an area of your life where you are acting according to your values? What personal strengths does this suggest you have?

_____

_____

_____

Think about areas of accomplishment or competence. Can you identify any areas of your life in which you've achieved some level of skill or competence? This didn't happen by magic—it came from practice, perseverance, and commitment.

Maya recognized that, although it felt overwhelming at times, she was actually managing to keep up her home, care for her two children, and go to work every day. She acknowledged that maintaining this balance—even if at times it felt as if she was not doing a very good job—was an important accomplishment, one that required a wide range of competence and skills. Ed recognized that he was a competent woodworker. He had earned this competence from hours and hours of working at his trade. He acknowledged that this had taken perseverance, patience, and commitment.

What is an area of competence for you? What skills do you have—abilities that may not have come completely naturally, but which you've had to work on? What personal strengths does the development of these skills suggest to you?

_____

_____

_____

Now take a look at the personal qualities you identified about yourself as you answered these questions. Allow yourself a moment to acknowledge your strengths and your resilience. How can you bring these qualities into your everyday life? What are some challenging situations you are currently facing where you can rely on these qualities?

_____

_____

_____

Be Grateful

There's an old expression that we really like: "Happiness is not about having what you want—it's about wanting what you have." Similarly, gratitude is wanting what you have. It's noticing and appreciating the things in your life—big and small—that add value and contribute to your well-being.

Maya reflected on what she was grateful for. She immediately thought of her children and her friends. She felt silly, but she was also grateful for the cup of tea that she enjoyed every morning. Ed was grateful that, despite his hand pain, he was still able to work on small woodworking projects. He also felt grateful for his car—especially when it was freshly washed!

There are many ways of cultivating and expressing gratitude. You may want to keep a gratitude journal. It's a wonderful way of reminding yourself on a daily basis of the good things in your life. You can also make it a point to let others know that you appreciate them—send a text or an email, or make a quick call. Gratitude is often contagious!

Think of one or two things in your life that you can be grateful for today. Write them here:

_____

_____

_____

Stop and Smell the Roses

When something good happens, pause, take notice, and enjoy it. Tell yourself, *This is really lovely* or *What a treat!* Try to take a mindful attitude toward life—be present for as much of it as possible. For example, I (Nina) try to make it a point not to eat my lunch in front of the computer. I want to pause and appreciate the taste of the food.

Think of an activity you'll engage in today that is pleasant for your senses—eating tasty food, listening to nice music, or walking in nature, among others. Pause during the activity and notice the pleasant sensations you are experiencing. Then allow yourself to appreciate them. Write down the activity you've chosen to appreciate. How did it go?

_____

_____

_____

Practice Mindfulness

As we saw in chapter 10, mindfulness-based skills are useful for dealing with the negative, demotivating thoughts and feelings associated with depression. In addition, mindfulness has been shown to be helpful in maintaining a depression-resistant life (Segal and Walsh 2016). When practiced regularly, mindfulness can also be an important part of a routine that contributes to deeper levels of happiness and well-being.

There are many ways you can incorporate mindfulness into your daily life. You can start by practicing the breathing exercise you learned in chapter 10. If you look online, you'll find many videos and apps to guide you through a variety of mindfulness exercises. Mindfulness programs—usually in person and group based—are available in many communities. One of the best mindfulness programs that we know of—one that's tailored specifically for people either struggling with depression or wanting to keep depression from coming back—was developed by psychologist Zindel Segal (Teasdale, Williams, and Segal 2014). As of this writing, his online course can be found at https://www.mindfulnoggin.com.

Like any type of activity that you want to incorporate into your life, you'll need to make a specific, doable plan to practice mindfulness. And like any type of skill, the more you practice, the more naturally it will come to you, and the more you'll benefit from it.

What would a good plan to add mindfulness to your life look like?

_____

_____

_____

Exercise Self-Compassion

Compassion is about being kind to oneself and others when faced with difficulties, failure, or mistakes. Multiple research studies have found a strong link between self-compassion and overall well-being (Gilbert 2017; Neff 2023).

Many of us have a very harsh and self-critical inner voice, especially when we think we have made a mistake or failed in some way. While we think that self-criticism will motivate us to be better, in reality it leads to a downward cycle of avoidance and depression (Neff 2023). Think about it for a moment—what happens when you are highly self-critical? Does it motivate you, or does it leave you feeling demoralized and inclined to withdraw and avoid? What about when you are kind to yourself? Research suggests that when we show kindness and compassion toward ourselves, we tend to feel better, we are more effective at facing and solving our problems, and we show greater patience and perseverance (Ewert, Vater, and Schröder-Abé 2021).

Practicing self-compassion involves recognizing your self-critical harsh self-statements and then consciously being kind to yourself. Here are some examples of compassionate messages you can practice giving to yourself:

- "You are doing the best you can."

- "It is normal to find this hard."

- "Many people struggle with this issue."

- "It is normal to make mistakes and sometimes experience failures."

- "Failure is how you learn and grow."

- "While not perfect, you are doing a good job."

- "Given everything that is going on in your life, you are doing well."

It can be helpful to think about how you would express compassion to a friend—and then direct those same compassionate statements to yourself.

Think of a situation where you tend to be self-critical. Now try to develop a couple of kind, compassionate statements that you could say to yourself. Feel free to use the examples we gave, or come up with your own. Write down the compassionate self-statements that you would like to use:

_____

_____

_____

_____

Next, close your eyes and imagine that you are experiencing the situation where you would normally be self-critical. Rather than your normal self-critical statements, imagine telling yourself

self-compassionate messages. Try talking to yourself in a gentle, kind, compassionate tone of voice. Really hear these messages. Pause for a moment. What did it feel like?

_____

_____

When you're having a tough day—struggling to face your problems, experiencing a sense of failure, feeling inadequate or incompetent—try very consciously to adopt an attitude of self-compassion. Be kind to yourself—see if it makes a difference.

Time to Say Good-Bye

Congratulations on making it through to the end of this workbook! We've covered a lot of ground together. We hope that you've been able to benefit from the behavioral activation strategies we've shared with you, and that you're feeling better than when you started. Life being what it is, you will probably hit some rough spots—we all do. But please try to remember the principles of behavioral activation—and keep on pressing forward. Behavioral activation won't make the rough spots disappear, but it will help you get through them.

As a good-bye, we wish you a happy, depression-resistant life, full of fun, meaningful activities, gratitude, wonderful relationships, and every good thing.

Acknowledgments

We would like to start by thanking the many clients with whom we've had the privilege of working over the years. These courageous individuals have been willing to share their stories and their problems with us—and in the process have helped us learn about the power of behavioral activation.

We were blessed with wonderful editors at New Harbinger—Elizabeth Hollis Hansen, Madison Davis, and Karen Schader. From start to finish, they were always available with helpful advice and support. Special thanks to Ben Swallow for his help with the diagrams and figures we used throughout the book, and for his helpful feedback on earlier drafts. Dr. Zindel Segal has been a longtime friend, colleague, and support to both of us. We very much appreciate his willingness to write the foreword to this book.

I (Nina Josefowitz) would like to thank my many students whose questions and curiosity helped me articulate the essence of behavioral activation. I would particularly like to thank two colleagues. Dr. Michael Rosenbluth gave me the push to submit the proposal and generously offered support throughout the process. Dr. Joyce Isbitsky provided thoughtful comments on many of the early chapters. The many clinical discussions throughout the years with both Michael and Joyce are reflected in this book. Lastly, I would like to thank my family, children, and grandchildren for providing love and balance to my life, and Novak Jankovic for everything.

I (Stephen Swallow) would like to thank my friends, colleagues, and students at the Oakville Centre for Cognitive Therapy for providing me with a stimulating and supportive professional home. To my family—Peter and Sarah, Ben, Wesley, and Liam, and most of all my wife, Karen—thank you for your patience, your love, and your encouragement.

References

Abildso, C. G., S. M. Daily, M. R. Umstattd Meyer, C. K. Perry, and A. Eyler. 2023. "Prevalence of Meeting Aerobic, Muscle-Strengthening, and Combined Physical Activity Guidelines During Leisure Time Among Adults by Rural-Urban Classification and Region—United States 2020." *Morbidity and Mortality Weekly Update* 72: 85–89.

American Psychological Association (APA). 2019. *Clinical Practice Guideline for the Treatment of Depression Across Three Age Cohorts*. Washington, DC: APA. Retrieved from https://www.apa.org/depression-guideline.

Bandura, A. 2008. "An Agentic Perspective on Positive Psychology." In *Positive Psychology: Exploring the Best in People. Vol. 1: Discovering Human Strengths*, edited by S. J. Lopez. Westport, CT: Greenwood Publishing.

Barton, J., and J. Pretty. 2010. "What Is the Best Dose of Nature and Green Exercise for Improving Mental Health? A Multi-Study Analysis." *Environmental Science and Technology* 44: 3947–3955.

Basso, J. C., and W. A. Suzuki. 2017. "The Effects of Acute Exercise on Mood, Cognition, Neurophysiology, and Neurochemical Pathways: A Review." *Brain Plasticity* 2: 127–152.

Beserra, A. H. N., P. Kameda, A. C. Deslandes, F. B. Schuch, J. Laks, and H. S. de Moraes. 2018. "Can Physical Exercise Modulate Cortisol Level in Subjects with Depression? A Systematic Review and Meta-Analysis." *Trends in Psychiatry and Psychotherapy* 40: 360–368.

Blankert, T., and M. R. W. Hamstra. 2016. "Imagining Success: Multiple Achievement Goals and the Effectiveness of Imagery." *Basic Applied Social Psychology* 39: 50–67.

Blumenthal, J. A., M. A. Babyak, P. Murali Doraiswamy, L. Watkins, B. M. Hoffman, K. A. Barbour, et al. 2007. "Exercise and Pharmacotherapy in the Treatment of Major Depressive Disorder." *Psychosomatic Medicine* 69: 587–596.

Cacioppo, J. T., M. E. Hughes, L. J. Waite, L. C. Hawkley, and R. A. Thisted. 2006. "Loneliness as a Specific Risk Factor for Depressive Symptoms: Cross-Sectional and Longitudinal Analyses." *Psychology and Aging* 21: 140–151.

Canadian Network for Mood and Anxiety Treatments (CANMAT). 2016. "Clinical Guidelines for the Management of Adults with Major Depressive Disorder: Section 2. Psychological Treatments." *Canadian Journal of Psychiatry* 61: 524–539.

Chekroud, S. R., R. Gueoguieva, A. B. Zheutlin, M. Paulus, H. M. Krumholz, J. H. Krystal, and A. M. Chekroud. 2018. "Association Between Physical Exercise and Mental Health in 1.2 Million Individuals in the USA Between 2011 and 2015: A Cross-Sectional Study." *Lancet Psychiatry* 5: 739–746.

Cuijpers, P., L. Wit, A. Kleiboer, E. Karyotaki, and D. Ebert. 2020. "Problem-Solving for Adult Depression: An Updated Meta-Analysis." *European Psychiatry* 48: 27–37.

Diener, E., and M. E. P. Seligman. 2002. "Very Happy People." *Psychological Science* 13: 81–84.

Ewert, C., A. Vater, and M. Schröder-Abé. 2021. "Self-Compassion and Coping: A Meta-Analysis." *Mindfulness* 12: 1063–1077.

Gilbert, P., ed. 2017. *Compassion: Concepts, Research, and Applications*. London: Routledge.

Hays, K. F. 2012. "The Psychology of Performance in Sport and Other Domains." In *The Oxford Handbook of Sport and Performance Psychology*, edited by S. M. Murphy. Oxford: Oxford University Press.

Herrod, J. L., S. K. Snyder, J. B. Hart, S. J. Frantz, and K. M. Ayres. 2022. "Applications of the Premack Principle: A Review of the Literature." *Behavior Modification* 47: 219–246.

Hirshkowitz, M., K. Whiton, S. M. Albert, C. Alessi, O. Bruni, L. DonCarlos, et al. 2015. "National Sleep Foundation's Sleep Time Duration Recommendations: Methodology and Results Summary." *Sleep Health* 1: 40–43.

Ingram, R. E. 1990. "Self-Focused Attention in Clinical Disorders: Review and a Conceptual Model." *Psychological Bulletin* 107: 156–176.

Josefowitz, N., and D. Myran. 2021. *CBT Made Simple: A Clinician's Guide to Practicing Cognitive Behavioral Therapy*, 2nd ed. Oakland, CA: New Harbinger Publications.

Josefsson, T., M. Lindwall, and T. Archer. 2014. "Physical Exercise Intervention in Depressive Disorders: A Meta-Analysis and Systematic Review." *Scandinavian Journal of Medicine and Science in Sports* 24: 259–272.

Kabat-Zinn, J. 1990. *Full Catastrophe Living: Using the Wisdom of Your Body and Mind to Face Stress, Pain and Illness*. New York: Delacorte Press.

Kanter, J. W., R. C. Manos, W. M. Bowe, D. E. Baruch, A. M. Busch, and L. C. Rusch. 2010. "What Is Behavioral Activation? A Review of the Empirical Literature." *Clinical Psychology Review* 30: 608–620.

Li, Y., M.-R. Lv, Y.-J. Wei, L. Sun, J.-X. Zhang, H.-G. Zhang, and B. Li. 2017. "Dietary Patterns and Depression Risk: A Meta-Analysis." *Psychiatry Research* 253: 373–382.

Lin, T.-W., and Y.-M. Kuo. 2013. "Exercise Benefits Brain Function: The Monoamine Connection." *Brain Sciences* 3: 39–53.

Malhi, G. S., E. Bell, P. Boyce, M. Hopwood, G. Murray, R. Mulder, et al. "The 2020 Mood Disorders Clinical Practice Guidelines: Translating Evidence into Practice with Both Style and Substance." *Australian and New Zealand Journal of Psychiatry* 55: 919–920.

Manber, R., and C. Carney. 2015. *Treatment Plans and Interventions for Insomnia: A Case Formulation Approach*. New York: Guilford Press.

Miranda, M., J. F. Morici, M. Belén Zanoni, and P. Bekinschtein. 2019. "Brain-Derived Neurotrophic Factor: A Key Molecule for Memory in the Healthy and the Pathological Brain." *Frontiers in Cellular Neuroscience* 13: 363.

National Institute for Health and Care Excellence (NICE). 2022. *Depression in Adults: Treatment and Management. NICE Guideline No. 222*. London: NICE.

Neff, K. D. 2023. "Self-Compassion: Theory, Method, Research, and Intervention." *Annual Review of Psychology* 74: 193–218.

Parikh, S. V., L. C. Quilty, P. Raitz, M. Rosenbluth, B. Pavlova, S. Grigoriadis, et al. 2016. "Canadian Network for Mood and Anxiety Treatments (CANMAT) 2016 Clinical Guidelines for the Management of Adults with Major Depressive Disorder." *Canadian Journal of Psychiatry* 61: 524–539.

Pearce, M., L. Garcia, A. Abbas, T. Strain, F. B. Schuch, R. Golubic, et al. 2022. "Association Between Physical Activity and Risk of Depression: A Systematic Review and Meta-Analysis." *JAMA Psychiatry* 79: 550–559.

Premack, D. 1959. "Toward Empirical Behavior Laws: I. Positive Reinforcement." *Psychological Review* 66: 219–233.

Richards, D. A., D. Ekers, D. McMillan, R. S. Taylor, S. Byford, F. C. Warren, et al. 2016. "Cost and Outcome of Behavioural Activation Versus Cognitive Behavioural Therapy for Depression (COBRA): A Randomized, Controlled, Non-Inferiority Trial." *Lancet* 388: 871–80.

Segal, Z. V., and K. M. Walsh. 2016. "Mindfulness-Based Cognitive Therapy for Residual Depressive Symptoms and Relapse Prophylaxis." *Current Opinion in Psychiatry* 29: 7–12.

Teasdale, J., M. Williams, and Z. Segal. 2014. *The Mindful Way Workbook: An 8-Week Program to Free Yourself from Depression and Emotional Distress*. New York: Guilford Press.

Torre, J. B., and M. D. Lieberman. 2018. "Putting Feelings into Words: Affect Labeling as Implicit Emotion Regulation." *Emotion Review* 10: 116–124.

Vrugt, A., and C. Vet. 2009. "Effects of a Smile on Mood and Helping Behavior." *Social Behavior and Personality: An International Journal* 37: 1251–1258.

Waldinger, R., and M. Schulz. 2023. *The Good Life: Lessons from the World's Longest Scientific Study of Happiness*. New York: Simon and Schuster.

Nina Josefowitz, PhD, is a clinical psychologist. In addition to her clinical practice, she teaches at the University of Toronto, and has offered training in North America, Asia, and Africa. She is author of numerous professional articles on cognitive behavioral therapy (CBT) and issues related to general clinical practice. Along with David Myran, she coauthored *CBT Made Simple.*

Stephen R. Swallow, PhD, is a clinical, health, and rehabilitation psychologist; and founder of the Oakville Centre for Cognitive Therapy, one of Canada's leading CBT clinics. In addition to maintaining an active clinical practice, he provides supervision to mental health professionals-in-training, and teaches CBT both domestically and abroad.

Foreword writer **Zindel V. Segal, PhD,** is professor of psychology at the University of Toronto Scarborough. He is coauthor of *Mindfulness-Based Cognitive Therapy for Depression* and *The Mindful Way through Depression.*

MORE BOOKS from
NEW HARBINGER PUBLICATIONS

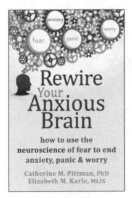
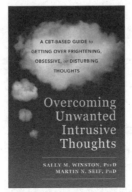
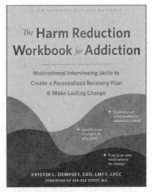
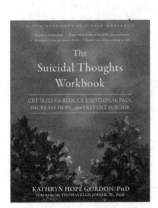
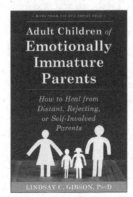
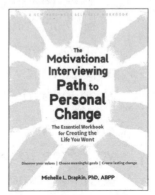

Did you know there are **free tools** you can download for this book?

Free tools are things like **worksheets, guided meditation exercises**, and **more** that will help you get the most out of your book.

You can download free tools for this book—whether you bought or borrowed it, in any format, from any source—from the New Harbinger website. All you need is a NewHarbinger.com account. Just use the URL provided in this book to view the free tools that are available for it. Then, click on the "download" button for the free tool you want, and follow the prompts that appear to log in to your NewHarbinger.com account and download the material.

You can also save the free tools for this book to your **Free Tools Library** so you can access them again anytime, just by logging in to your account! Just look for this button on the book's free tools page.

+ Save this to my free tools library

If you need help accessing or downloading free tools, visit **newharbinger.com/faq** or contact us at **customerservice@newharbinger.com**.